# It's Just a Headache

C.A. Rothermund-Franklin

It's Just a Headache

**Authors Note**

THIS BOOK DOES NOT offer medical advice, a cure, suggestions for treatments nor does it imply in any way the reader follow or attempt the experiments the author describes in the prose that follows. This migraine memoir recounts the author's experiences, efforts, trials and errors to manage headaches through the course of a lifetime. Seek professional medical assistance from a board certified neurologist to treat your migraines. Commiserate here.

Events described are based on the author's memory. Effort was made to remain true to factual depiction of situations. The names of persons in this book were altered or changed out of respect and privacy of those involved.

Cover image

Modified from: A face turned away, suffering acute pain.
Lithograph by P. Simonau, 1822, after C. Le Brun.

**It's Just a Headache**

**lost to a migraine**

**C.A. Rothermund-Franklin, PhD**

*~For Mom~*

When long naps in the dark came

We didn't know

It's Just a Headache

## CONTENTS

It's Just a Headache

# PROLOGUE

I WOKE FROM A fitful sleep. The throbbing increased as conscious awareness of my surroundings began to form. It was dark, sometime in the middle of the night and I was cold. I moved to turn over and find the blanket, but the pain intensified. It wasn't going away.

I took a deep breath, lifted my head from the pillow and turned my shoulders in preparation to rise from bed. I pushed up with my arms and sat upright then lowered my legs to the floor. They trembled as the carpet rubbed like course sandpaper against the bottoms of my feet. As I stood, my head swirled and body tilted forward. My eyes wouldn't focus in the dark. Bile crept up the back of my throat as my stomach bounced against my insides. I needed to get to the bathroom and fast. The dim glow of the nightlight placed over the vanity led the way. I stumbled across the room and grabbed hold of the doorframe to steady my gait. The muted shadow of my reflection appeared then swayed in the mirror. Beads of cold sweat formed on my forehead then began their slow trickle down the sides of my brow as my hands searched in darkness for the refill packet. *Where was it?* I thought in frustration while I rifled through the drawer. *I should keep these ready for times like this.*

A wave of nausea overcame me. I gripped both sides of the sink and leaned forward as the reflexive force of dry heaves took over. Sweat poured down the sides of my face with each empty purge. My breath hard and fast, I dropped my forehead on the faucet between each cycle and splashed water on my face to cool down. The spasms subsided, and my attention returned to the drawer. My fingers bumped then grabbed the familiar dual cylinders and case. Finally, there it was. *Snap!* It was inserted and ready to load. I needed a steady hand to use it. This part was never easy. I shook with anticipation as the cold, round barrel pushed against my flesh. I turned my head away and squeezed my eyes shut. *No, wait,* I remembered. *I needed to sit down.*

I slid the shower curtain aside, folded my legs and sat on the floor next to the tub with my arm propped on the edge. *Pop!* It was in. A bead of blood followed the sting, and a new a rush of nausea returned. I regretted sitting so far away from the toilet and sink. The tightness squeezed my throat first then sunk into my stomach and intestines before making its loop up towards my neck. It slowed down as it moved to my head. The sharp tingling chased away the warmth from the dry heaves, and a chill took over. *Why didn't I bring the blanket?* I thought as cold from the tile floor wicked up and into my body. I laid my head on the arm propped on the tub, careful to avoid the tender needle prick from moments ago, drew my knees up to my chest and waited.

It's Just a Headache

**Part I**

**More than a headache**

It's Just a Headache

I REMEMBERED THE FIRST time. I worried if my hair was styled perfectly, was anxious about the clothes I wore and if they met the strict standards of the cool girls and in a panic if my face was breaking out. Chin buried in the nape of my neck, I looked up only to keep from tripping on any of the new strangers. As I passed one guy, my arm accidentally brushed his shoulder. I pulled away quickly and found a seat across the aisle as his eyes almost met mine then darted away. I slid all the way in then turned my head to stare out of the window.

The bus jerked forward, wheels crackling on loose gravel, as a swirl of orange dust and faint smell of sulfur from the exhaust trailed behind us. After a few moments to work up courage, I peeked over my shoulder. The guy had turned and was facing forward into the aisle. He caught me looking, stretched his hand out and introduced himself as Jerry.

"You must be the girl from Florida," Jerry said as he backed up slightly into his seat when our hands touched briefly.

"Yes, I'm Christy," I replied nervously pulling my sweaty hand back quickly but perking up at the sound of the home I'd left behind.

"Well, there's not a lot to do around here, but after school, some friends and I play basketball if you want to join us", he continued. "And, my dad's the preacher if your family needs a Church," Jerry finished as he turned back towards the inside of his seat, his voice trailing off as if the last part of his introduction about the invitation to his dad's Church was versed.

Jerry's thick, southern drawl made it hard for me to understand what he said, and he didn't look me in the eye when he spoke. I pretended to get something out of my backpack and moved towards the middle of my seat, so I could peek over at him during the rest of the bus ride to school. He fidgeted, stared out of the opposite window then jumped up and raced down the aisle the minute the bus pulled into the school.

My family moved to Andes Ridge a month prior. Most people migrate south to Florida, but our family was opposite. We left sunshine, palm trees and fishing in the Gulf of Mexico in our boat for a small town in the Appalachian Mountains when my father retired. I came home from my last day of middle school and found empty boxes stacked in my bedroom waiting to be filled and a for sale sign on the boat.

"We'll take it out this weekend one last time," daddy said, puffing the last bits of tobacco from his Pall Mall before he flicked it down to the ground and snuffed it out with his boot. "I have to make sure everything works before anyone comes over the buy it," his voice trailed and a dissipating cloud of smoke followed behind him as he walked away towards the back yard shed to finish packing up his shop tools.

I was up before momma or the sun. Daddy already had the boat hitched, and we left early for Ruskin, a town a few miles south of Apollo Beach. We stopped on the way at the convenience store and picked up ice and sodas for the cooler then docked the boat at Simmons Park. Once launched, I coasted slowly through the tidal zone to make sure we wouldn't bottom-out on any sandbars then pushed it to full throttle, and we distanced ourselves from the shore. We made it to the Sunshine Skyway Bridge, and I dropped anchor next to a crusty pylon to fish as cars passed like tiny toys nearly four hundred feet above our heads. That was the last time I would ever see the bridge before a barge brought down the southbound lanes and claimed the lives of thirty-five people a few years later. We fished until the day grew late, and daddy ran out of cigarettes. Momma got worried if we stayed out past dark, so I pulled anchor while daddy got the Evinrude started. I cut the biggest wake I could as I drove us back to the dock.

The boat was heavier than I'd ever felt it as I cranked it onto the trailer. Once I had it all the way up, daddy got out to check to make sure I had it secured properly. He stood for a minute, looking over the trailered boat from one end to the other, finished his Pall Mall from the spare pack he kept in the car and then threw the smoking remnants of the cigarette into the water. We pulled in the driveway at home just before dark. Someone interested in buying the boat had called while we were gone.

***

The afternoon bus dropped off Jerry and me across from the elementary school. The basketball court lay in front of the street alongside a creek near the gym. From the distance, I saw two figures. One was a dark-haired medium-build female who sat on the corner of the court while the other girl practiced shots at the net-less hoop. Kara stood as we approached and offered a half smile as she reached out her hand to introduce herself. Sissy offered only a brief hello as she ran by chasing down a missed shot, then turned and bounced the ball towards me to join in.

I dribbled and took a three point shot from the left corner, which missed and rebounded hard to the right. Jerry made a quick save and scored a one point layup. Kara stampeded in for the recovery, spun past Jerry almost knocking him over and then easily landed a two pointer. The ball didn't even touch the barren metal ring when it went through. I recovered the ball as it landed in the grass and rolled down towards the creek then passed it to Sissy who dribbled around Kara, faked a shot Jerry tried to block, and then made a two pointer. We continued our scrimmage for about a half hour, breaking the ice of

11

nervous introductions until Sissy suggested we head up the holler to the restaurant for a cold soda and peanuts.

A bell on the door clanged when we opened it to enter the restaurant. To the immediate right, an empty two seat table sat next to the window looking out to the road. Along the side walls were shelves stocked with grocery items, convenience store sundries, candy bars, gum and peanuts. A coffee counter stretched across the back of the restaurant, overlooking the grill, with cigarette ash trays placed in front of each seat. Spires of smoke drifted up from lit cigarettes as customers sipped on crew coffee and caught up on town gossip. Across the restaurant and against the back wall past the pool table sat the juke box. The sound of country music playing in the background was in competition with the hum of upright coolers as the volume drifted through clouds of stale cigarette smoke. Jerry left to grab each of us a cold soda while I fed quarters into the pool table and set the rack. With a hard snap against the front corner of the triangle, the balls were set tight for the start of our game.

"Who wants to break?" Kara asked as she picked out her favorite cue. Sissy looked over to Jerry with a sideways smile as he returned and handed her a soda, like she already knew they'd be partners. I broke since I was the

guest and sunk the lucky solid followed by three more.
Sissy was a good basketball player, but she wasn't very
good at pool, and Jerry couldn't carry the game on his
own. Kara and I cleaned up the pool table three out of five
games straight. We ran out of quarters and since it was
getting late and about time for dinner, we called it a night
and decided to head home.

"You live up Ridge Road holler, right?" Jerry asked as
he held the door for us. Kara exited first.

"See ya," her voice trailed as she intentionally bumped
Jerry goodbye with her elbow and sped off. Sissy smirked
at Jerry as she passed him in the doorway, her eyes queued
and then jerked past him like something was wrong, then
she left quickly without saying anything. I meandered out
last and into the gravel parking lot close to the road trying
to see where Kara and Sissy had gone so quickly. I sensed
Jerry already knew where I lived. He gestured for me to
follow him as he walked around the side of the restaurant
and showed me a hidden alley that led up through some
shrubs to Ridge Road, a shortcut home.

The good thing was I could get home from the
restaurant taking the alley behind the building. It was a two
minute walk to my front door taking the shortcut up the
holler. Every route to get somewhere in our small town

was up a holler. The problem was none of my new friends were in any of my classes at school. Kara was older than the rest of us, but that meant she could drive. She had a car although technically it belonged to her father. She was a reserved, quite type and didn't say anything about school. I assumed she had already graduated. Kara didn't have a job at least, not one she got dressed up and went to work at. She took care of her father, a retired coal miner who never left the house. Kara ran the errands, picked up his pharmacy orders, groceries, his cigarettes and beer. I never knew about her mother. She never mentioned one.

Sissy was in eighth grade which was part of elementary school. Tall with early developing feminine curves and anime-like green eyes, she could have passed for older than twelve. Her medium brown hair fell thick around a wide, smooth skin face. It didn't look like she ever had acne before. She dressed in big city clothes and always wore the newest styles. As a first string forward on the basketball team, she was the star player, and everyone on the team knew who she was, but no one seemed to be friends with her. She talked a lot about her games, practice and shopping for new clothes.

Jerry was fourteen and a year ahead of me in High School. He parted his dark brown hair on the side, which was common for guys at the time. He hid behind the low hanging part that covered his forehead and eyes. When he tossed his head back and ran his fingers through his hair, a handsome face was fully exposed. His jaw was firm, sharp and tapered up to a perfectly shaped set of lips that he held parted all the time, like he was ready to say something but afraid to speak up. He was tall, for an average fourteen year old, and dressed in freshly pressed clothes with button down shirts always tucked in with the top button secured. His medium-tan skin tone matched his brown eyes. Of his four brothers and six sisters, Jerry was the youngest of the brothers and the one that stood out. He was the reserved and quite one in the chaos of his overcrowded home. Jerry's father worked in the coal mines during the day and ministered the congregation on weekends. That was where he learned to play. Even though Jerry never had formal music lessons, he was a talented guitar player in the Church band.

Jerry wasn't on the school bus every day, but I looked for him, and if he wasn't I assumed he got a ride with one of his older brothers or sisters. I didn't have anyone to catch a ride with but was stuck on the bus for my transportation to and from school. I always got off the bus after school in front of the basketball court in the afternoons to check if any of my new friends were there. Sissy had practice three days a week after school in the gym next to the basketball court. She was usually there, but other times, her older brother picked her up. He was her chauffeur for shopping and club events. Other times, I thought he was checking up on her because he never said anything to us. He would park on the edge of the lot, backed in, so that when Sissy hopped in and they left, he spun out and kicked loose gravel at us. But, I liked it best when it was just Jerry and me.

Getting to know Jerry was like having to be reacquainted every time we met. It was awkward enough to leave me guessing if we were just friends or kids experimenting with our growing curiosities. When it was just the two of us, I think he let me win. We'd play a few games, get past the nervousness of being alone for the day, and when we were sure no one else would show, we'd sometimes follow a trail down the embankment under the bridge and sit on the ledge of the abutment where no one could interrupt. Jerry always seemed to be holding something back.

When Kara showed up to join us after school, she parked the car near the teacher's parking lot, where visitors were supposed to park, and waited for us to show up. She was there the day it was raining. It was pouring when Jerry and I got off the bus. We both made a beeline dash for Kara's car. Jerry jumped in the front seat, and I took the back. We waited, thinking the rain would let up and also, to see if Sissy would show.

"Let's go!" Kara blurted out as the rain pounded, and more dark clouds rolled in over the ridge to the west.

"Maybe we should go home?" I questioned as Kara peeled out of the parking lot heading north up the ridge.

"I've got something for you two," Kara said as she pulled a can of beer out of her purse. She handed it to Jerry, then reached in, grabbed another and twisted her arm behind her head to hand it to me. I hesitated then took the can from Kara and sunk back into my seat as Jerry popped the ring on his and drank half of it before I could say a word.

Kara sped up. I was nervous, but I didn't want to say anything. The wipers could barely keep up with the pounding rain against the windshield as we raced north up the ridge. I looked down at the beading condensation on my can of beer, working up courage then saw Jerry slam the rest of his, crush the empty can in his fist, roll down the window and toss it out. A rush of wind and rain blew in with the opened window, which startled Kara and made her overcorrect on a narrow curve. She hit the brakes, and the car spun sideways then flew off the road. We came to rest in muddy gravel. The force of deceleration pushed me against the door and the can of beer flew out of my hand and landed at my feet. Luckily, I hadn't opened it yet. Realizing the car was upright and we were all OK, Jerry and Kara burst out laughing. Then, the blue lights came on behind us.

Silence fell inside the car. It wasn't funny anymore. The cruiser sat behind us for what seemed like hours then the sheriff got out and approached the driver's door. The rain had let up some, but drizzle poured off the brim of the sheriff's hat as he tilted his head and glared inside the car at the three of us and asked, "have you kids been drinking?" I was sure he saw the spin out, tire tracks or maybe even Jerry when he threw the empty beer can out of the window. *We'd be on our way to jail.* I thought as my heart raced. My throat was too tight to answer the sheriff's question. Kara jumped in confidently, like nothing had happened and answered, "No sir, I'm driving my friends' home from school."

The sheriff reached his hand up and tilted back his hat, so he could lean closer into the partially opened window to look deep and hard to see what was inside the car. Kara crushed out the cigarette she was smoking in the ash tray then cranked the handle to completely roll down the window. Smoke billowed out as Kara leaned over, covering her purse and the other beers, to allow the sheriff's head partway inside the car to perform his inspection. I had pushed my feet forward to lean back and shoved the unopened can of beer I dropped under Kara's seat. It was safe and out of sight. I was stiff with fear as the sheriff's eyes probed the insides of the car and our guilty conscious. Then he stood and straightened his hat and glanced up briefly as a heavy rain shower started again. "Ya'll need to head on home now, there's a storm," the sheriff warned, satisfied he'd done his job. As he turned to head back to his cruiser, rainwater had already pooled in the brim of his hat, and a trail spilled behind him as he hurried away.

No one said a word as Kara lit another cigarette then started the car and drove down the ridge, slow and cautious, as the rain beat hard on the windshield. I was too afraid to reach down to pick up the beer still shoved under Kara's seat. I held it secure with my foot while we were driving, so it wouldn't roll out. Kara stopped to drop me off at the end of the driveway in front of my house. As I grabbed my backpack and got out of the car, I reminded her of the beer under the seat. She nodded and acted as if she wasn't worried about it, flicked the cigarette she was done with out of the window and then took out another one and lit it. I turned to say bye to Jerry, but Kara had already rolled up the window and started to drive away. I was relieved the crisis was over, but that would change when it happened for the first time the following week.

I wasn't popular, but I was a model student. I never missed a day at school and earned good grades without much effort. I spent my free time at the basketball court or the restaurant with Jerry, Sissy and Kara then went straight home and got my homework done after dinner. I minded my parents and took care of my chores. I was never a problem child. The day it happened started a little off. I woke up feeling tired like I hadn't slept well. My lower back hurt and on the right side of my head, there was a slow and steady pulsing. I'd never had a menstrual cycle before. I was thirteen years old, so it was about time for it to start. In a hurry to get her makeup and hair done for school, my older sister gave me a maxi pad and told me I might need it. I shoved it down to the bottom of my backpack, flung the strap over my shoulder and headed into the kitchen to grab something to eat before school.

Mom had made toast and eggs for breakfast, and I felt a little better after I ate but didn't mention the headache. Who tells their mom anything? I was off to the bus stop with the maxi pad hidden safely in my backpack. My head still hurt, but I figured it was nothing and would go away.

The sulfur exhaust hit me before the bus came to a full stop. It was much stronger than I remembered it before, and the smell made my stomach turn. It continued to follow me as I climbed on and scanned the seats as I walked down the aisle to see if Jerry was on the bus. I was relieved I didn't see him, since I wasn't really feeling up to socializing anyways. I found my usual seat, slid all the way in then reached up to the window and lowered it to let in some fresh air. I rested my head on my backpack, which I'd placed on my lap, to hide my eyes from the light as the bus rumbled on towards school. By the time the bus pulled in to let us off, the sun was up. I wasn't feeling any better, so I waited for everyone else to get up out of their seats and down the aisle before I started my exit. I needed to hold onto the backs of the seats for support. Once I stepped off the bus and into daylight, the morning sun felt like knives stabbing in my brain. I ran to get inside the school building and out of the light. I was feeling dizzy once I got inside, so I went straight to class.

The classroom was empty as I opened the door and entered. I dropped my backpack on the floor with a thud and plopped down in my seat in the front row. I pulled out my books for the class, spread them opened in front of me on the desk then lowered my head and shielded my eyes from the overhead light with my spiral notebook standing upright. I rested quietly for a while before other students, and then the teacher arrived. All we ever did in first period English Lit class was sit motionless and stare down at our desks. I got started early. I moved my pencil every once in a while to make it look like I was making progress. The teacher never left her desk in the front of the classroom to check on us. She poked her head up above the book she was reading, scanned the room for erect pencils and heads and no gum chomping as the sign we were doing what we were supposed to. Thankfully, that was the case since all I'd done was drawn a few chicken scratches on the paper in front of me for fifty minutes.

The second period bell rang like a hammer against the right side of my head. I flipped my book closed, grabbed my backpack and went to stand. My legs trembled as I stood and arms shook as I lifted the meager weight of the book off the desk. My next class was only a couple of doors down, so I stopped at the fountain to see if a sip of water would make me feel better. My hand shook as I twisted the knob and drank at least a pint of cold water. It was more than I had planned, but I must have been thirsty, and the cold water felt good rolling down the back of my throat. The tremors had moved up my arms by the time I sat down in second period class in sync with a pounding in my head. The overhead lights were even brighter than in English Lit class and focusing on the teacher, sitting at her desk only a few feet away, proved difficult. She had a fuzzy halo surrounding her. I fidgeted nervously at this new symptom. I opened and closed my eyes several times to try and focus, but the haze wouldn't go away. I turned my head from side-to-side, but everything I tried to focus on was surrounded by a halo. I blinked faster, but that made me dizzy and the teacher suspicious why I was giving her double eyed winks. Sweat broke across my forehead as a wave of nausea made me gasp out loud which signaled the attention of my classmates. I straightened my back and shoulders against the chair and for a moment, I thought everything was OK, I could handle it. I closed my eyes in an effort to gain composure, but my head started to spin, and I felt like I was falling over as waves of nausea followed excruciating pain on the right side of my head. Embarrassment built. I feared I would vomit right there in front of everyone all over the desk, my shirt and the floor. Classmates that only knew me as the quiet student who sat in the front row began to whisper, "What's wrong with that girl?"

I had to get out of there. The light filtering in through the windows was killing me, the sound of the door opening and closing was explosive, and the smell of teenage girls drenched in perfume and boys' cologne was suffocating. I couldn't see. My eyes were open, and I struggled to focus, but everything was surrounded by halos. My head was exploding from the inside. I gathered myself, rose from the chair and asked the teacher if I could be dismissed from class to use the restroom. She saw I was in distress and quickly slid the hall pass across her desk. I grabbed the pass, made it to the door of the classroom, closed it behind me and exited into the hall. To my right were rows of gray lockers stretching for what seemed miles to the end where the restrooms were located. I took in a deep breath for the long walk to the girl's bathrooms. As I exhaled, the hall began to spin, slowly at first and then faster as I took the first step forward. I reached my hand up, tried to grab onto the lockers for support then everything went black.

The school nurse refused to accept my answers. I hadn't taken anything, and I wasn't pregnant, either. Her probing questions made my head hurt even worse. I didn't know how I got to the principal's office, but she kept staring at me, tapping her pen on some papers spread out across the desk in front of her, waiting for a big reveal. I slouched in the chair, trying to disappear. I was embarrassed. My head felt like it would explode if a spark would ignite the quite crackling polyester pill balls between the cushions I was sinking into. I didn't know what was happening while I waited for my parents to come get me like a silly lost child at a department store. I heard them talking in the next room before they came in to escort me out. Being a new kid in school, I didn't have a prior history but then, I'd just made some. I was sent home in the care of my parents after a search of my backpack revealed a soda, bag of peanuts and a hidden maxi pad. My mother kept peeking over her shoulder to look at me shielding my eyes from daylight as we drove home. She didn't say anything, but a curious look on her face made me anxious I was in trouble once I felt better. When we finally arrived home, I ran to my room, went directly to bed, curled up and cradled my head in my hands.

News travels fast in a small school especially when it's a new kid who passed out from a drug overdose. That was the story by the next morning. The whispers, darted eyes and heads turned away suddenly when I looked were proof positive most of the school thought I was a druggie. I wasn't friends with anyone at school. I hadn't been there long enough. I kept my head down and went through the days' classes looking up only to follow instructions from my teachers. Not much changed in how I went about a typical day.

I didn't see Jerry on the bus ride to or from school for the next several weeks. I figured he got a ride with his brothers or sisters. He'd done that before. I didn't want to face him and have to talk about what happened in the hallway. I went straight home and got busy on my homework and reading books. It's not like that was a bad thing after all. I was a good student even though the rumors were otherwise. Aside, I was afraid another one of the headaches would come.

It was months later when Jerry came to the door of my home after school. I heard the knock but was in my room when my mother answered.

"Ma'am, can Christy come down to the basketball court?" Jerry asked in his coy, polite southern drawl, staring down at his feet the whole time. I looked out of my bedroom window and saw Sissy nervously pacing at the end of the driveway. The basketball was tucked under her arm as she kicked around gravel in what looked like a new pair of Converse high toped shoes. She glanced up and saw me. I waved at her from my window, and she raised the basketball above her head, gesturing me out. I threw aside the book I was reading, grabbed my shoes and put them on. I almost tripped over my feet as I ran outside. In such a hurry to get back to my friends, I hadn't bothered to tie them.

Sissy bounced the ball hard and fast as we walked down the holler towards the basketball court but refused to look at me. I kept glancing over to her, expecting the ball to come firing in my direction at any moment. Jerry stared at his feet as he walked, like he usually did, but I saw the crooked smile of contentment on his face. He was happy the three of us were together. Finally, the uncomfortable silence between us broke.

"What have you been up to?" Jerry asked as we stopped just before the bridge to cross over the creek. I turned to face Jerry, just as he swooped his head and eyes down to the ground. Over his shoulder, the trail that led under the bridge to the abutment we sat on was visible. Sissy was staring at it.

"Well, I've been trying to stay out of the halls at school," I answered as my faced blushed with embarrassment. "I checked out some books from the library and was reading to keep myself busy."

"Oh yeah, what have you been reading?" Sissy butted in sarcastically and asked. I wasn't really sure what Sissy meant by her question. From her tone and how hard she was slamming the ball against the asphalt as we walked, I sensed she was mad. I didn't know what Sissy knew. It had been such a long time since I'd seen anyone. She *was* in middle school, and I assumed rumors from high school didn't drift that far. I didn't think Jerry would say anything, and Kara didn't seem to care much for her. Sissy probably knew nothing about the spinout and the sheriff's stop and search of the car on North Ridge Road—that was months ago. But, from the sound of Sissy's question, she was irritated and wanted to know something more than about what books I was reading.

"Well, today, I was reading Aldus Huxley when you guys came up to the house. My English teacher said it was a good book for students who want to study medical science," I explained, answering only the obvious question as we arrived at the net-less hoop.

"I read Vogue and Seventeen," Sissy chimed in; not happy with the answer I'd given but taking over the conversation abruptly. "I'm going to UT when I graduate. I'll get a scholarship to play basketball and become a model, too," she continued as we stopped and both turned towards Jerry, expecting that he'd say something about what his plans were. It was his turn to share. After all, he had started the uncomfortable conversation. Jerry had never opened up about what his future plans were, and I was curious. I hoped we shared some common interests outside of the rectangular basketball court where we met after school.

"Are we playing or what?" Jerry blurted out then leapt forward and grabbed the ball out of Sissy's hands then stormed towards the goal for a one point layup as if the ongoing conversation about books, reading and what we planned for our futures had never taken place.

It's Just a Headache

***

The next headache was similar to the first but this time, I didn't pass out. It came like a lightning bolt out of nowhere except, there was no storm to give forewarning. My monthly cycle was close to start, and my lower back ached. The sunlight hurt my eyes, and I could see stars like I'd hit my head. The pain radiated in pulses from the right side just above my eye. The waves of nausea were the worst. It felt like I would throw up at any moment. It was hard to sit through classes when the headaches came. Bile seeped up the back of my throat, and the sick feeling made me afraid to eat anything. I was pencil thin through High School because I couldn't eat and often, wouldn't eat because of the headaches. When they came, I clenched my fists, bit my tongue, held my breath and any another pain-transfer method a thirteen year old could think of to try and channel the throbbing pain away. None of those worked.

I hid them. I didn't want my mother or anyone else to know. Back then, we didn't want to stand out with special needs. Fitting in meant we were like everyone else. We didn't have problems, and I didn't want to be a problem or a disappointment since there were rumors. I wanted my friends and those at school to accept me as a normal person not some clenched fisted, tongue-biting, breath-holding special child with a suspicious mother in-tow. The whispers had faded since the first episode when I made a fool of myself passed out in the hallway. I was not going to let that happen again. But, Jerry noticed when I wasn't myself. I couldn't hide the pain from him even though I thought he wasn't looking me in the eye.

I'd skipped Church services since Kara, Jerry and I had our run-in with the law and since I'd passed out in the hallway at school. It seemed like most of the uncomfortable feelings had passed and things were getting back to OK especially since Sissy and Jerry had come up to my house with an invitation to play basketball. I thought I'd surprise Jerry and show up at Church. I'd wear something nice, too. My older sister stared at me suspiciously as I pilfered her closet for a more mature dress that Sunday morning. I didn't normally wear girly clothes, but things were changing. I found a navy blue and white dress with semi-mesh netting at the neckline. It was a Florida-type dress but was more form fitting than any I had on my side of the closet.

I slipped into the Church from a side door greeted with pleasant purse-lipped smiles as I scanned the pews for Jerry. *He must be up front with the band,* I thought. I was a little uncomfortable, feeling like a new outsider all over again as I made my way towards the back where Jerry and I usually sat. I'd walked to the Church alone that morning in my big girl dress. When I'd attended services before, Jerry came up to my house and walked with me. This morning, I was on my own continually looking down at the provocative mesh hung low around my neck pulling up on it every few minutes like something I didn't have yet was going fall out.

I looked down at my neckline, wrinkled now from the abuse and turned to find my seat in the pew and there was Sissy with a surprised look on her face.

"Hey, what are you doing here?" Sissy greeted me as I motioned, politely for the seat next to her.

"I thought I'd come to services today," I answered, taking in the visual of how mature and classy she looked. Sissy's designer dress matched the teal hue of her eyeshadow. Her hair looked as if she had only moments before stepped out of a salon, after hours of work and bickering stylists made sure her hairdo was perfect. A thin-banded, gold watch around her wrist and a necklace hung appropriately with a tiny cross accentuating the low cut V-neck of her dress. She could have easily passed for older than I was.

"Your dress is pretty," I complimented Sissy as I sat, small and ordinary next to her then crossed my legs in proper lady-like fashion. I reached for the song hymnal, grabbed an extra one and passed it to her. She nodded and looked down as she began to fumble through the book to find the song page. The music director approached the pulpit and asked the congregation to bow for opening prayers. We lowered our heads, but I peeked and saw Sissy check me over. My borrowed dress was from the sale rack at Kmart. My hair wasn't styled in any special way. I wasn't allowed to wear makeup yet, and I didn't own any fancy jewelry.

The choir began, and my nervousness eased. I saw Jerry playing the guitar, swaying back and forth in rhythm with the music looking down at his feet like he always did. Once the choir finished opening hymns, Jerry slipped away from the band, snuck around and emerged from the back of the Church to join Sissy and me. I straightened my back and drew in my arms tight as Jerry sat to my right. Sissy fidgeted with her watch, crossed her legs to the left then to the right several times during the sermon then stood straight up and raced out of the building without a word the second after closing prayers concluded.

"I should have let you know I'd be here today," I apologized to Jerry as we rushed to follow Sissy outside. We rounded the corner of the exit doors to see Sissy's brother was waiting to pick her up, puffs of smoke drifting out the driver's side window of the Lincoln Town Car. Jerry lagged behind me but as I stepped off the sidewalk to catch up, it was too late, she had already jumped in, shut the door, and they sped away.

"She must have basketball practice or something," Jerry said in an anxious tone I'd never heard in his voice before. I made an about face, turned and started to march back home, regretting that I'd shown up at Church that morning in the first place. Jerry followed behind me. "I can't walk with you today, but can you go somewhere with me next Saturday?" he asked. Anxious to separate myself from the uncomfortable situation, get home and change out of the too-low cut neckline I was wearing, I didn't ask where but agreed to go with Jerry and continued to hurry towards home. I'd made it to the first turn when I saw Kara driving towards me. She spotted me, slowed momentarily and waved, then sped up and drove on towards the Church. I stopped and waited for a minute to see if she'd come back then turned around to retrace my steps to look up the street towards her. Kara had pulled into the parking lot. Jerry emerged from inside the Church, jumped in the front seat of Kara's car, and they left.

There wasn't a lot to do in a small town. Outside of school, scrimmage at the basketball court, soda and peanuts at the restaurant and maybe a game of pool, Andes Ridge didn't offer many amenities. I debated through the next week whether I should keep that promise to meet Jerry on Saturday. I didn't know what he had planned, and he hadn't been on the bus for me to ask him. I wanted to meet up after school at the basketball court to find out, but my mother had my sister and I busy that week at home. She has us clean and organize our room, arrange our dressers to separate clothes we didn't wear any longer then help sort through closets in the house to decide what to keep, what to toss and what to send for donation. By late Saturday, I'd earned a break to go out. Not sure what to expect, I threw on a decent pair of jeans, T-shirt and straightened up my hair then headed over.

I found Jerry and his older brother Lance finishing their Saturday evening chores inside the Church. "You two can head out, and I'll finish up here," Lance said as I offered to help empty trash cans from the Bible study rooms. "We have men's fellowship meeting tonight. I have to stay late," he continued. Timid in the presence of his older brother, Jerry tilted his head down, submissive, as we moved to the door. We exited the Church and found Kara parked in the back waiting for us.

"You're going, too?" she asked in a disappointed voice when she saw me approach the side of her car. Jerry got in the front passenger seat, and I slid into the backseat. We could have walked. It was only a few blocks away.

We entered the barn from one of the front doors partially opened into a room filled with people and music. In the back and on a makeshift stage, fashioned from fresh-cut hay bales, pine two-by-fours and used pallets, a band played contemporary Christian music. It was the type full of energy with electric guitars, bass and drums. The music was exceptionally loud as if we were at a concert rather than a religious gathering.

"I'll be right back," Jerry said as he left for a moment to go up to the stage and talk with some of the musicians. Jerry disappeared into the crowd then Kara, who had fallen silent since we left the parking lot at Church, turned towards me.

"I have to go out to the car," she snapped, then turned to retrace the path we had only moments before entered from. Abandoned by my hosts, I took in the magnitude of the room. I recognized some of the people as regulars from Church, but others I'd never seen before. Clumps of people were gathered in social groups strew throughout the room as the music played raising the adrenalin of everyone present. My heart pounded in sync with each beat as the music grew louder then a man entered the stage, took the microphone, and the band silenced. He roused the audience with religious phrases, and a call-response ensued. Each time the man quoted a phrase, the crowd grew louder and more excited. I was slowly back stepping my way to the exit when Jerry returned.

"Where's Kara?" he asked.

"She went back to the car," I yelled, barely able to hear over the volume in the barn. "I think she forgot her cigarettes," I continued as people slithered around us.

Jerry leaned in close enough that I felt the warm condensation from his breath on my ear and said, "We have to get closer to the stage." For a moment, I caught the smell of beer but wasn't sure where it came from. More people had entered the barn since we had got there. The crowd was packed in tight around us. Jerry grabbed my hand, and we squeezed through the crowd up to within a few feet of the stage, so I could see what was going on. The air was stuffy, and it was a lot warmer that far into the barn, like the pens where cattle were corn fed to fatten them up before they were sent off for slaughter. The exit doors to freedom were far behind me now. I wasn't able to see the floor of the stage, but I saw the man reach down, and before I knew it, he held a snake above his head as the electrified crowd cheered.

My heart stopped then dropped into my stomach when the snake writhed and turned its head towards the man holding it up for the crowd to see. I thought it was a fake. It couldn't be moving like that. I broke my grip from Jerry's hand and made a bolt for the door. Jerry followed and caught up with me just as I made it to the exit. He reached out for my hand, but I pulled back.

"I have to go," I said, breathing hard trying to catch my breath. "I need you to meet me at the restaurant after school next week."

The bell clanged as Jerry opened the door. He pulled out the chair for me at the two seat table at the restaurant. I stared out the window up the holler towards the basketball court while he went to get sodas. The hum of country music played in the background, and the smell of grease fried hamburgers mixed with cigarette smoke filled the air. Jerry returned and sat our drinks on the table, already beading condensation from the heat filtering in through the window. We'd met to say our goodbyes because my family was moving back to Florida. We talked about school coming up, what we planned to do until then and when we might see each other again. Jerry had never been to the ocean. I asked him to come visit me in Florida, but he turned his head or darted his eyes when I pressed the idea. I scribbled my address on a napkin then slid it across the table. He fumbled with his soda and then wiped the water off his hands before he took the napkin, folded it and placed it neatly into his front pocket. We promised to write each other, call if we got a chance and shared a moment where our eyes met.

***

I scooped two heaping spoonful into the glass of water and stirred. Glen already had his spinning in a vortex. "You have to mix it really fast before you drink it," he warned. I turned mine a couple more times and tipped the glass for a sip. The smell of stale yeast invaded my nostrils as the liquid rolled towards the end, but I stopped at the last minute. I had to do it. Glen already had his gone. The insoluble chunks had stuck to the insides of the glass when I took the first sample sip. I used the spoon to push them back down into the yellow mixture and stirred again. They weren't dissolving. With a last quick swirl, I slammed a mouthful spilling some down my chin in haste to get it over with.

"This stuff is awful," I said while gagging the last of it down. "How do you drink this every day?" I asked Glen while I used the sleeve of my shirt to sop the spilled liquid that was running down my chin.

Brewer's yeast was one of many health craze supplements in the early 1980's. We purchased one and two pound jugs of the powders to mix tablespoon heaps into water and then drank it under the assumption we were doing good for our bodies. The health benefits aside, the yeast-water colloid tasted like cardboard and smelled like pond scum. It made my stomach hurt, too. The soy lecithin powder wasn't that bad. It mixed with water better but still tasted odd. After learning to drink Brewer's yeast, I had the spin and gulp method down pat. B-complex vitamins came as pills although, some were rather large, but I'd learned that good health came with sacrifices. Gagging on putrid mixtures and choking on horse pill sized vitamins were a small price to pay in an effort to avoid the headaches. That was the idea.

I met Glen at the restaurant where we both worked. He was a swing-shift cook, and I washed dishes on swing and was a cook on graveyard shift. He was into health food, exercising and read a lot of books. The nutrition guru we all went to for advice, he talked about starting a business in health and fitness where he could help others reach their well-being goals which he would have been good at it had he ever given it a go. Glen was the epitome of perfect health. He was a stout, blond-haired, blue-eyed German full of energy and enthusiasm. He never broke a sweat in the sweltering kitchen, kept his cool even when customer orders backed up the window and kicked out food faster than any other cook. The waitress liked him and, the best part was he was single.

I showed up in South Florida at the age of eighteen. It was my first taste of independence. After my family returned to Tampa from Andes Ridge a few years previously, I moved across the state to live with my older sister. She helped me get a job at the restaurant, and we rented a two bedroom apartment located only three blocks away from the beach. My room had an oversized walk-in closet and patio doors that led out to a pool. I parked my red, ten-speed bicycle on the patio, dropped my two bags of clothes in the corner and slept on the floor since I didn't have the burden of furniture yet. When I wasn't at work or sitting through classes at the Community College, I lay out in the loungers at the pool, studied or hopped on the bike and rode along A1A, a highway that parallels the Atlantic Ocean on the Southeast coast of Florida. The trek took me from Ft. Lauderdale north towards Boca Raton and a few times I rode farther, so I could get past the crowded beaches. Most of the coastal real estate was privately owned by hotels, condos or timeshares which were all blocked off and not accessible. Public access was few and far between. If I wanted a quite spot, I had to ride several miles north almost to Delray, but it was worth it.

I lifted and carried the bike since the tires dug in when I pushed forward on the handlebars. Passing through the narrow opening between the mangrove shrubs, the white sand beach and ocean emerged on the other side as the hum of traffic disappeared behind me. I secluded the bike from obvious view in the foliage, untied my shoes, took off my socks and placed them behind the front wheel then headed down to the surf. The sunbaked sand seared my bare feet as I exited the cover of shade. I picked up the pace and ran toward the breaking waves. I could feel the oceans pull once my feet hit the cool wet, sand. I stopped, stood for a minute, curled my toes in the softness under them and adjusted my backpack. The gritty, shiftiness gently exfoliated my soles as I waded out into the shallows.

Up the beach and in the distance, a couple meandered along the shoreline. They stopped and knelt down every few moments. I guessed them tourists hunting for seashells, out to see what treasures the Atlantic Ocean waves had dropped off for them to steal away. I eyed them for a few minutes, to see where they were headed, so I'd know where I wouldn't go.

The secluded beach was overtaken by high rise hotels and condos. That was what shielded it from the ever present hum of traffic on the other side--even if that meant the beauty was pillaged by tourists and time share vacationers. The tiny sliver of public access I was allowed reminded me of my place, also demarked by the signs delimiting how far I could wander. But, it didn't matter. The oceans roar was constant, and the waves pushed a breeze onshore in both directions.

The couple came closer. They were as averted to me as I was to them. I knew that because their backs were turned, and the No Trespassing sign stood between us, but as they drew closer, I could see more clearly what they were doing. They were hunting seashells but not finding suitable ones. For every handful scooped, they were tossed aside. Not satisfied, and at the end of their privileged beach, they turned and started their stroll back. Relieved the couple was gone; I scanned the narrow beachfront for a shaded spot to settle in. I wasn't there to take anything away. I was there for therapy where I could read, write in my journal and breathe in the warm, salty air. It made my head feel good.

The headaches clustered around my monthly cycle. When they came, I had to power through them because there was my share of rent, utilities and cable with MTV to pay. Living on my own was expensive especially if I wanted perks like music video on TV which at that time was the only channel on cable that made its expense worth paying. I had to work even if I had a headache. When the headaches came, I hid out in my walk-in closet. Instead of using the closet for normal things like shoes and clothes, I had it setup with a thick blanket for a mattress and pillow where I could escape into total darkness away from the light and noise that made the headache worse. Dark and quite was the key to getting through them. There was a pattern. I knew the headaches would come a few days before my cycle. That was blackout time. I never planned anything then.

"You need vitamins for your brain," Glen leaned over and whispered in my ear, lingering intimately close to my face. The clean smell of shower gel hung in the air behind him, momentarily wiping away my stench. Glen fell back into his chair then glanced at his watch. Dressed in jogging shorts and a sleeveless T-shirt, he was ready for his morning run. I leaned back in my chair, struggling to maintain composure from a headache that had started the night before then reached up to rub my forehead. My fingers slid across stale fryer grease that had seeped into creases etched from a too tight chef's hat. We were at an employee meeting that morning, and I was eager to head home afterward having finished a graveyard shift. I had to get through this meeting, ride my bike back to the apartment, shower and then crawl into my safe, dark and quiet closet until it passed. I wasn't in the mood for socializing when my head hurt, but Glen noticed the times when I didn't feel well and wanted to help.

I jumped in the shower the minute I got back to the apartment. As steam leached out grease from the night before, I thought about what Glen said. Maybe he was right about the vitamins. If something was missing, that could be what caused the headaches. I'd never thought much about what I ate and how it affected how I felt. From what Glen said, when he changed his diet and started taking vitamins, he went from tired and sluggish, to lean and full of energy. I grabbed my meals between shifts. Working at a restaurant meant we ate mistakes or plates rejected by customers. If the waitresses didn't want the rejected food, they brought the plates back to the cook's window, and we sat them aside in the kitchen and smuggled them to whoever wanted or needed a free meal. Though we got an employee discount to order food during our breaks, most of us scrounged customer rejects freeganstyle. That meant I might eat fried chicken one night, because the customer wanted white meat and the plate went out with dark, or a warmed over Reuben sandwich because the customer didn't want the type of cheese it had. I never knew what I'd eat, other than it was a free reject plate of food.

Glen never ate rejects. He didn't eat fried foods, limited his meat intake, consumed copious amounts of fresh vegetables and didn't drink anything that had caffeine. He took the employee discount and designed and cooked his meals for breaks, so they were low salt, low fat and attractive to the eye and palate. The meals Glen made for himself on breaks turned out looking like something off the cover of those health food magazines. As Glen explained, most of our food had too much fat, salt and fillers which leached essential vitamins and minerals from our bodies. With a few modifications, one could be on the road to better health, and it all started with what we ate.

Stress, grease and sweat from the night before swirled and then disappeared down the drain as I shut off the shower. I was clean, but tired and my head still hurt. I crawled into the closet, pulled the door closed and slept the rest of the day. Sometimes, I could sleep off the worse part of a headache especially if I was dead tired and it was quiet and dark like in the seclusion of my tiny closet. Because I alternated between swing and graveyard shifts through the work week, I never adjusted to a stable sleep pattern, but that was only part of life's irregularities.

It was dark when I woke. My stomach growled and head swirled as I opened the closet door and crawled out to stand. Hunger pangs reminded me I hadn't eaten since the day before. I grabbed my clean uniform out of my clothes bag in the corner, got dressed and headed out to the patio to jump on the bike to head into work early. I poured a cup of coffee at the waitresses station then slipped back into the kitchen to pilfer reject plates for something to eat before my shift started. There was Glen, looking fresh and energetic at the end of his eight hour work day. You would have never known by looking at him that he had just finished a dinner rush shift in the grease pit.

"Are you eating that?" he interrupted. "Those heavy carbohydrates are just going to bog you down," he went on as I grabbed a hot beef potatoes and gravy. I looked down at the plate of food I'd chosen. To my left sat a two egg breakfast reject, but the hash browns were burnt, and the eggs were rubberized. The hot beef plate was the only edible choice even though the top layer had gravy skin, and the potatoes had dried out. I could scrape away the bad parts and lob some butter on it to soften it up and make it edible.

"I'll take care of it and cook you something healthy," Glen announced as he flung a clean towel over his shoulder and turned towards the grill. Suddenly embarrassed at the fact I ate rejects, I turned away to hide my face, blushing as I took the too-old-to-eat hot beef potatoes and gravy and dumped it in the trash in the dish room. I traded my cup of coffee for a tall glass of ice water and disappeared to wait in the employee break room to see what I'd get for dinner.

Glen introduced me to the health and nutrition stores in town. I took him to the pool, beach, and we sat on the patio of my apartment while I listened to him talk about his home in the Midwest. I'd never traveled that far north before, but I could almost smell the dried corn dust swirling in the air as Glen described how combines harvested the fields in late summer. Row after the row, green turned to gold then farm equipment lumbered out of their barns and toiled for days on end until all the fields were done, as Glen explained. Just like we stayed out on my patio past sunset, until the yellow turned to reds on the horizon, and then the parking lot lights took over for the rest of the nights when we stayed up on our days off. What meant most to Glen was health and fitness. He believed almost any illness could be cured if we changed our diet and committed to an exercise plan, and I believed him. Glen helped me setup a diet plan to get rid of my headaches. I scrapped pretty much everything I normally ate, gave up caffeine for plain water and fruit juice, added fresh fruits and vegetables and took vitamin supplements as part of my daily routine. It wasn't tough to stick to the plan, when Glen was around, which was most of the time. While our relationship grew into an engagement, months passed, and pounds of Brewer's yeast, soy lecithin and vitamins gulped down didn't stop the headaches even after we moved into an apartment together and became vegetarians. Something changed, but it wasn't planned. What stopped my periods also stopped the headaches.

It's Just a Headache

\*\*\*

My foot sunk then disappeared with a crunch as I trudged forward with each step. A stiff wind blew loose hair across my forehead. I tried to tuck the strands, but my gloves were beaded with ice crystals. The soggy glove soaked my hair and I ended up shoving matted, wet clumps under my hood as ice melted behind my ears.

"I can't see the broad side of the barn," I yelled over to Glen, laughing at the corny joke I'd made then the wind threw a swirling tuft of snow in my face and took my breath away. It wasn't funny any longer. I pulled down on the bottom of my coat, stretched tight around me, to keep the horizontally flying snow from seeping into my midriff. My shoes were wet, and I couldn't feel my toes. Glen continued on to the pole shed. He was dressed appropriately in a warm down jacket and watertight boots. He hopped through the knee deep drifts and made sure to steer clear of the grain bin and barn where the wind blew showers of loose snow from the edge of their roofs. In my naivety, I was drawn to them for shelter and pummeled as I tried to follow.

"It's called whiteout," Glen yelled, standing under the shelter of the shed. No, whiteout was a bottle of liquid we corrected mistakes on typing paper when we used old-fashioned typewriters. This was the coldest I had ever been. What was a mistake was letting a 20-year old, improperly dressed, pregnant girl wander around in a blizzard on a farm in Nebraska. I needed to get back to the house and warm up.

Glen and I packed up our apartment in South Florida to head for family friendly living in Nebraska once the stick turned blue. We rushed the wedding, so I'd still fit into the dress. During the drive north, it started to get cold in Tennessee, and that's where we stopped and bought a coat. I didn't own one because it never got that cold in Florida. I chose one that was my normal size so it would still fit after the baby was born. We spent everything both of us had saved on the wedding then used the money we received as gifts to rent a U-Haul and put gas in the car for the move to Nebraska.

February was not the best month to arrive looking for a home, six months pregnant, unemployed and a U-Haul trailer crammed with everything we owned, so we moved in with Glen's parents on the farm until we could find jobs and our own place. We unloaded our belongings into the barn to store temporarily and lived out of a few bags of clothes in Glen's old bedroom at the farmhouse. All the stories Glen had told about the flat, wide open space and tall grass prairies in Nebraska were true except, I wasn't expecting it to be so desperately cold. I missed my home back in Florida, lounging by the pool, warm breezes and the sun. It was a twenty mile drive from the farm into the city which was a long way to go to look for work and a doctor we could afford to deliver the baby. The only good thing was the headaches were gone. If there was a transient cure, it came with pregnancy and the bitter cold of Nebraska winter. I'd not suffered a headache since I missed my period, and the pregnancy test we had rushed out late one night in a state of panic to buy from the drug store showed a bright blue streak for positive.

It's Just a Headache

***

I stared out the windows looking for any sign a car might pull into the parking lot from the Interstate. It was after 2am, and my last customer had shuffled out more than an hour before, leaving the usual 76 cents behind. That was the leftover change I received for a tip after the two dollar cash out paid for coffee. The late shift waitress went home early at 10:30 and left me, the cook and dishwasher to another slow weeknight on graveyard at the restaurant. It was tough to find help willing to work overnights, but I was lucky to get the job. I searched for over a month and was desperate. During the interview, the manager rustled nervously through his paperwork, and I squeezed sideways in the booth because my belly wouldn't fit sitting forward. I didn't mention the eight months pregnant when I applied. He must have felt sorry for me because I was wedged in for the entire hour interview. He hired me for a part-time starting position. My assigned shift was graveyard, but I taped a handwritten note next to the time clock with my name and phone number on it to let the other waitresses know I was available for call in's especially if that meant I could work swing shift. I was willing to come in to work at a moment's notice for those. Swing shift was the best time to make money because that was dinner rush and when families came out to eat. Other women, mothers especially, were the best tippers, and I played on their understanding of my condition. I waddled up to their tables bellied-out and back bent, so I would look miserable and ready to deliver. They felt sorry for me, and the money rolled in.

"Do you have your hospital kit ready?" Anna announced as she approached the cook's window, leaned against the edge and dropped her customer order book as it fell and slapped against the counter. She twisted sideways facing me and tilted her head. Her eyes rolled down to look me over, taking in the girth of my situation, as her fingernails tapped a dull thud against the greasy surface waiting for my response. She pursed her lips and squinted, but gentle, upturned curves at the corners of her eyes gave way to only a soft grimace of disapproval. Her attention quickly tracked back to her own business where she ripped off her customers order sheet then snapped it on the cook's wheel and started to tray up an order that was ready. I looked at Anna like a pregnant feral cat, shown up at the door last minute ready to birth a hungry litter. I didn't know what this kit was I should have ready to go when the baby was born. I inched towards Anna, timidly, and shoved another customer order under the clip of the wheel and started to search the window to tray up my order that should have been ready for delivery. The ticket was there, laid out with my waitress number light on the way the cook's let us know our order was ready, but I couldn't find any of the food for the ticket.

*Where was it?* I thought as irritation built. *Was everything missing for this order?* I panicked and crushed the ticked in my hand.

"You're order's right here," Anna butted in. I turned to see Anna's head tilted slightly to the side, eyes squinted and lips pursed with nails tapping fast and hard on the counter. "I trayed your food order, she explained as her voice lowered in volume and intensity. "It's ready to go." She reached around me and flipped my waitress light off then walked away toward the salad station.

I got those call in's to work swing and struggled late into my pregnancy to heave loaded trays on my shoulder. I needed the money and to make a good impression, so the manager would consider taking me on swing shift after I had the baby. Anna was there most nights I was called in on swing to work and took pity on the young newcomer, cleared the herd at the cook's window so the bellied-up one could get through and even followed me out to the tables a few times to help unload food from the heavy trays. She made sure I took my breaks, ate a decent meal and helped me get my end of shift work done. We always left work at the same time, even if that meant Anna waited around until after her shift ended. She acted like she was busy doing other things, but I knew she was waiting for me. Our store was tucked behind the onramp of Interstate 80, and employees parked behind the store in the back lot.

Anna's voice was commanding, but the spirit of a kind woman hid behind dark brown eyes that could see right through you. When she decided something needed done, you followed, moved aside or Anna took you under her wing. She was a born leader, teacher, mentor and benevolent dictator, but I was a long way from ready to fledge. She moved to Nebraska only a year before I did. Anna was a single mother, alone with three babies, a few bags of clothes and had started out in a room at the women's shelter. The Church outreach counselor met Anna at the shelter and took a photo of her and the kids then used it as a promo print on flyers to help raise money. They were the face of hope on donation containers that supported the women's shelter for many years. Anna started with nothing, but she was determined.

"I start classes this fall," Anna exclaimed as she raised her arms, lifted her head and broke into a victory dance next to the break table where I sat rolling silverware. "I got a scholarship. It's all paid for!" she continued. Anna's infectious enthusiasm couldn't be contained. Setting my envy aside for the moment, I was happy for her and wanted to jump up and give her a big hug, but that wasn't going to work. My belly wouldn't let me get close enough and aside, Anna's was a strong woman. I wouldn't risk compromising her command in front of all the other girls on shift.

Anna had everything going on. She had her own place, a decent car and was starting college the coming fall semester. I admired her. She was independent, mature and patient, especially with me. When the baby was born, I lay in the hospital, my feet freezing, thirsty for a soda which the hospital wouldn't give to new mothers and a slight throbbing on the side of my head I hadn't felt for close to nine months. Then, visiting hours rolled around. Anna came in the room with a devious smile, sent the nurse back to her station and pulled the hospital kit out of her purse.

She had stashed in her oversized bag a pair of warm socks, a cold soda and a chocolate candy bar which was exactly what I needed but didn't know enough ahead of time to bring.

I went home from the hospital with the baby and a pounding headache. I told the obstetrician before he signed my release forms that my head hurt, but he said it was because of stress and hormone changes. He recommended I take a Tylenol and said I'd feel better after a few days, but I knew differently. The headaches that had disappeared for the nine months I was pregnant were back with a vengeance.

***

"If you sit in the front row, the professor will spit on you when he lectures," Anna said holding back a smirk as she turned, trying to hide her face from me as she bent down to pick up her bag.

"That's not true!" I said shaking my head in disagreement as Anna burst out laughing. I rubbed the side of my hand across my brow. It suddenly felt like something was on my face. Anna grabbed her briefcase, stood and brushed her hair aside as she slid the strap on her shoulder.

"I have seminar. I'll see you later tonight when you drop off the kids," she announced, still grinning over the spit remark, then turned and headed toward the Arts and Sciences building. I gathered the notes I was studying and placed them into the book, careful to mark the page I'd left off then put them into my backpack and glanced up to the Bell Tower Clock. It was a few minutes before 2pm, time to head down to the University Library to my work study job for the next three hours before I needed to pick up the kids from afterschool care. Anna's daughter babysat the kids while I worked night's waitressing. They attended the same elementary school where an afterschool daycare was located on the premises. I dropped them off early weekday mornings at 6am, picked them up at 6pm and then took them to Anna's before I went to work at the restaurant for a dinner rush shift. They spent most weekends with their dad. I had that time open to work, study or get out with the girls to have some fun.

Glen and I called it quits after eight years of struggling. Married too young and stuck in a cycle of unfulfilled expectations, I rented a two bedroom apartment, packed a few bags of clothes and left one day when he was at work. I didn't want a lifetime hauling trays on my shoulders as a waitress. I'd always planned to continue my education. Anna was working on her graduate degree when I started college. She was my motivation as an example that I could do what she had already done. If she could go to college and complete a degree raising kids on her own, so could I. There were plenty of excuses I was making as to why I had not already taken the steps to get back in college and move forward; kids, work, money, and time, but all these were lame reasons for not getting my act together. Anna didn't let anything stand in her way. She met every challenge thrown at her no matter what it was, and that included dealing with headaches. There were plenty of obstacles to overcome being a single mother. The responsibilities of kids, work and college aside but we looked out for each other. I didn't have any family in town. Anna and I checked in on each other regularly to make sure everything was OK.

There were several messages on the answering machine. I still hadn't returned Anna's calls. It was late in the second day of a headache, and I'd been out of bed only to use the bathroom and take sips of water. Turning my body hurt, moving my arms was excruciating, and breathing felt like it further inflated my head with pressure. It was one of those explosive headaches that made me want to find the highest building and dive to the concrete below to escape the endless grip of pain.

"Bam, bam, bam...Christy...are you OK?" Anna shouted as she pounded her fists on the door. Curled in a fetal position, head cradled in my hands, the banging noise woke me in a sudden jolt. I wasn't expecting anyone. "Christy, are you there?" Anna's voice resumed with more urgency. She must have seen my car in the parking lot. I had to get up and answer the door. I uncurled, and my legs dropped to the floor.

"I'm here Anna!" my voice cracked as I struggled to speak rounding the corner towards the front door. My body shivered as a cold chill seeped through my pajamas. I unlocked the door as Anna rushed in.

"I was worried sick! You didn't answer your phone!" Anna's said with a sigh of relief.

"It's a bad headache. I was going to call back," I explained as my voice shook while I headed to the couch where I could wrap up in a blanket. Like hers, Anna knew I got the headaches, but they weren't always that bad. The ones that sent me to bed, curled up into a ball in an effort to shut out the world and ignore the phone for days on end were rare. Going for almost two days without a check in was unheard of and warranted an in-person well-being call. When these explosive headaches came, I had to escape, find an exit from light, sound and get into my quiet place where I could fall asleep, and when I woke, maybe it would be gone. This headache was nonstop for two days. Some of them were like that.

"I've got something my doc gave me. You take one to see if it helps," Anna said as she pulled a prescription bottle out of her purse. My stomach turned with preemptive nausea as Anna shook out a small, tan pill and handed it over. I hadn't eaten, but this medicine was destined to become my first sustenance in two days. In a futile delirium of pain, I resisted at first. It wasn't right to take a medication not prescribed to me. I didn't have my own doctor because I didn't have insurance. But, I needed both and trusted Anna. I gave in quickly and swallowed the pill down with a sip of water then lay back on the couch wrapped in the blanket.

"It takes a while before it works. I'll leave you alone now, but I want you to call me tomorrow," Anna insisted as the crinkles of worry turned to gentle, upturned curves at the corners of her eyes. She knew the headaches didn't like company. She left and I promised to call first thing the next morning.

I fell asleep quickly after Anna left. Her visit in itself brought some comfort even though I knew that getting through the headache was just a matter of time. It was a few hours later that I woke in darkness. My heart was racing, and I was drenched in sweat still wrapped in the blanket on the couch. It felt like thousands of tiny needles were stabbing into my skin. My stomach was knotted in cramps and bile seeped up the back of my throat. Pain from the headache was spread across my forehead, and the urge to vomit was overwhelming. I started to unwrap from the blanket, but as it touched my skin, it felt like fire pushed the needles further in. I dropped my legs to the floor to stand but they collapsed, limp and weak under the weight of my body. *What have I done!* The panicked thought raced through my mind as I remembered the tan pill. *I'm going to die!* I decided as I dropped to my knees and crawled across the living room floor, holding back the urge. Before that was going to happen, I needed to get to the bathroom to throw up.

***

Lessons learned the hard way were best. Mistake was a fine teacher. That was how the old saying went, but when it came to headaches that made me want to jump head first off tall buildings, all bets were off. When I swallowed a drug that wasn't prescribed to me, I wasn't afraid. The tears were from the bulging pain in my head, not fear. Once the pins and needles, trembling and dry heaves hanging over the toilet were over, I never knew if it was from the ergotamine or part of the headache.

There was a state of pain I had grown sickly accustomed. The headaches had reached a new level. For a while, I thought I'd get used to them or they'd get better on their own. Then an explosive headache would bring me to my knees, not able to stand, focus or function. It wasn't possible to hide a headache like that if I was at school, work or out in public. I'd always thought of myself as tougher than that. The demands of kids, school and work came first, not pain, but I didn't know when a headache started, how bad it would get. There was no way to know.

*Professor, please excuse me while I stumble out of class in the middle of your lecture. I'm dizzy, can't see straight and might vomit in the doorway on the way out. Oh, and if you believe this, it's just a*

**69**

*headache.* The insane thought raced through my mind sitting in an hour and a half physics class while the pain in my head continued to intensity. The tingling on the right side of my head had started early that morning. I took the first BC with breakfast which consisted of coffee and a bowl of cereal with the kids before we left home. It wasn't any more or less of a stressful day than usual. The kids were ready to go on time, and no one had any pressing issues. After I dropped them off at before school daycare, I headed on to campus. It was still dark when I made it to my first class, and by then the tingling had turned to painful pressure. I took another BC. Sometimes, a second one would take the edge off.

The sun had come up while I was in my first class, then when I left the building to walk to physics, the first light of day hit my head like a hammer and sent shooting stars into my visual field. I stopped at the water fountain in the hallway and forced down the third BC just before class started. My stomach rumbled as I settled into the seat. Students filtered in and chatted, shuffled their books and notes while we waited for the professor to arrive. Only two more classes to go and I'd be on my way to work study at the library where it was quite. I could get some rest there. The room went silent as the professor entered the lecture hall. My heart raced with a wave of nausea as I lifted my head towards the podium. Every time the professor spoke, which was nonstop, it felt like my eyes bulged out. I scribbled nonsense in my notebook, so classmates wouldn't notice the shaking that had taken over my hands, the tears welling or beads of sweat on my forehead. I glanced up at the clock, over and over a dizzying number of times, silently praying for the class to hurry up and end.

*If we could enter a time warp, class would be over by now,* I thought, trying to forget the pain in my head and bond with the lecture as I counted my breaths in an effort to hold back the urge. What I really wanted was to bolt in a straight line vector for the door. I needed an escape from the prism of pain I was trapped in. Finally, class ended. I exited staring down at my feet, taking careful, measured steps. I was afraid I would fall. The halos were everywhere, around everything I tried to focus on. I ignored them as I turned and disappeared behind the building and threw up where no one could see.

BC power was easy to take. It was finely crushed aspirin and caffeine. They fizzed up when I took them with soda which made the taste less bitter. When the tiniest sign of a headache came on, I unfolded a BC and tapped the powder onto the back of my tongue. Even though they didn't work, I took more than the maximum dose hoping they might help. I could maneuver the packet of BC powders with one hand. I unfolded the rectangular envelope with my thumb and forefinger, tapped the dusty powder onto my tongue using my pinky and washed it down with the soda I was holding between my middle digits, all without spilling a single grain of BC or drop of soda. I tried acetaminophen but was afraid if I took many they would harm my liver. Aside, they didn't help the headaches. Over-the-counter allergy medicines either made me drowsy or did nothing and left my head hurting. I fell back on aspirin and BC's because I thought they were safe despite the fact they made my stomach hurt, but I was already accustomed to the nausea that came with the headaches. What helped when a headache came on was a dark, quite place to wait it out until it went away. It came down to a matter of time, but I had to take care of my kids, attend classes in college and go to work. I found a near perfect solution in the basement of the University Library.

Work study was a mecca of escape from the stress of undergraduate classes and the headaches. I worked in the underbelly of the University Library where books were born. This was before computers took over, and students relied on printed forms of information to help them learn. I checked in new arrivals, much like a nurse might wrap a wristband on a newborns arm. I placed the magnetic strips inside new books as they were brought into the library.

Unlike the upper, public floors with full-length windows designed to let in ample lighting, the basement of the library was dimly lit, kept cool and dry to preserve the delicate book pages. The smell of fresh acid mingled with musty as new books continually cycled through to replace the old ones. Upstairs, the hum of whispers contrasted to a deafening silence in the basement. Only an occasional shuffle of footsteps indicated one or two of the staff was present downstairs. New books were catalogued according to their International Standard Book Number, ISBN, and assigned a Dewey Decimal Number for entry into the University Library according to the book's subject. Then, we hid the magnetic strip inside the book's binder, so they would ping a detector at the library exit, if it wasn't discharged at the checkout, and stamped the library catalogue details on the front and back covers to match the index information. Once the new book was processed, it was placed on the away cart destined for the upper floors and its final shelving location. That was the last time we saw them.

I loved it there in the underbelly surrounded by the task of delivering new books into the world of our library. Just as the nurse might pause for a moment to feel the soft folds on a baby's arm as she fastened the wristband, I paused with each book as my hands searched for its center. Sometimes, bumpy glue held the binding, but with others, a smooth stitching of cotton string weaved through the pages. Each book was bent, gently at the center, to ensure I didn't damage the binding, to insert the magnetic strip, so it was hidden for its lifetime. It was a manual process that only human hands could perform. I longed for the content held within the pages of the books I processed, but that wasn't my job. My part was brief. I ensured the book's life began with a hidden magnetic strip, was stamped with the library catalogue number and was placed on the away cart, so it was shelved properly upstairs in the light. But a few times I stopped and opened a book to browse and read a few pages. Strange covers hid fantastic stories. There was never enough time to follow them through to their endings. The away cart waited, and the next book needed processed.

Library science was an evolving discipline, and I considered it an option as an undergraduate degree. The quite work environment was an escape on the days my head hurt. The midwifery of books was a way to explore the world in the safety of the library cradle. It was possible to remain on campus those days when, otherwise, I'd never have been able to when a headache came on. The books I helped birth are long replaced by electronic versions or retired to dusty piles. My job at the University Library didn't pay much. It was minimum wage, and I was awarded only a few hours each week of financial aid work study, but I got to choose the hours, which made the job a perfect fit for my schedule. I worked there through my undergraduate career until I headed off to graduate school.

"You missed lab meeting this morning," Dr. L. scowled, his arms pinned tight across his chest, and his brow crinkled in anger as I cowered in late at 10:30.

"I had trouble getting out," I answered apologetically lowering my eyes and backpack to the floor then kneeling to sit submissive to his barking complaints. His bitter tone and the fact that he was waiting for me indicated that any answer I gave was not going to be good enough. I was on my second of three graduate rotations, and this one wasn't going well. The project was micromanaged, the mentor and I didn't bond, and I was having a lot of headaches since I'd joined the lab two weeks prior. I heard that Dr. L. was like this, but I had to have three rotations completed as part of the program, and his lab was working on a good project, even though he was a real pain. Since I had joined his lab, Dr. L. had decided to babysit every step I took and watch over my shoulder every moment of every day. He was attached to my hip, and it was driving me crazy. Trying to learn anything from the rotation with a lab mentor constantly breathing down my neck was not possible. I woke that morning to a pounding headache, took a BC and spent the next hour in the bathroom hung over the toilet. As I looked up at Dr. L., his lips pursed and squinted eyes waiting for my explanation, I wasn't willing to share anything with him. I wanted to get this rotation done and moved on as quickly as possible.

I chose my rotations so the third one was where I'd remain for my graduate program. My third and final rotation would land me in Dr. K.'s lab. As Vice Chair of the Department, Dr. K. was a mature, well-seasoned and supportive mentor who understood how to develop a graduate student. I would learn leadership, organization and discipline skills but most importantly, I'd be working in a lab under the mentorship of a person I respected. While the mentors had a meeting to bash the year's group of incoming graduate students a bit before deciding who they'd each keep, I was absolutely sure my second rotation would be a no and prayed Dr. K. would take me on.

Graduate school in the biological sciences was a full-time commitment. We worked under the guidance of our mentors in the lab on a research project and attended the required graduate courses. These typically took two years to finish. Once the coursework was done, a clock started ticking to complete the comprehensive exam. We were given one year to compose and present a National Institutes of Health grant to our graduate committee. This was to prove our fitness for PhD candidacy. If we passed comprehensives, an additional one to two years in our mentor's lab was needed to work on experiments in order to publish at least one peer-reviewed paper and compose our dissertation. On rare occasion, a graduate student might finish in four years. Most of these were the MD-PhD students in a hurry to get back to their clinical training. The rest of us had to think about post-doctoral fellowships. Getting done in five years was the goal we worked towards. A post-doctoral fellowship could last for several years, and usually, one was not enough. It was common in research to have multiple before setting off into a career. With the prospect of a meager graduate student stipend, the next five years working endless hours in the lab and five or more years in post-docs, I showed up for the first day of my third rotation.

"What project do you want to work on?" Dr. K. asked hastily, briefcase in hand and looking down at his watch as he hurried out of his office on the way to a meeting. His patience ended before it began as he continued through the lab and out the door. I started to open my mouth to answer just as the main lab door clicked closed behind him. Suddenly confused about what I was going to say, I turned and saw Andy, the lab technician, holding back his laughter.

"You're on your own here," Andy said, as his attention returned to his notebook. "I'm heading over to do some cell culture later if you want to come along. And, I need to get some samples setup for apoptosis assays if you want to help. It's up to you," he finished, still grinning over my failure to climb the first baby steps in the graduate student learning curve.

This was a complete one-eighty from Dr. L.'s lab where I had just finished a painful rotation. There, every move I made was supervised, instructed hand-held and watched over. I was going to like it here and agreed to follow Andy over to the cell culture facility since I was still a little rough on how to grow mammalian cells and needed to learn the technique. Apoptosis, or programmed cell death, was what really sparked my interest. Killing cells by convincing them to commit suicide was what apoptosis was all about. This altruistic pathway was how damaged cells made the ultimate sacrifice. In a normal cell, if something went wrong, the cell killed itself in a clean, organized and highly controlled fashion. The suicidal mess would not threaten the well-being of the entire organism. In the case of cancer, what we found most of the time was that the cancer cells had turned off apoptosis. Cancer didn't let cells commit suicide. Cancer cells were greedy, aggressive, self-centered entities that didn't care about the organism. They lived for themselves and in the process, the organism suffered.

Death was default. Those of us who worked in apoptosis knew that. Death was necessary for life, even at the level of single, individual cells. Normal cells were in an uphill struggle, ever on the verge of death at a moment's notice. The signals to remain alive must continually feed into a cell otherwise, it died. That was the normal way of things. When the signal to live ceased, for whatever reason, be that physical injury, detachment from the matrix or damage to the DNA that could not be repaired, the cell turned on its suicide program and death occurred.

When Spock gave his epic line, *the needs of the many outweigh the needs of the few or the one,* at the end of the movie Star Trek 2, The Wrath of Khan, in those last moments before he died, he was letting Captain Kirk know he was willingly to accept his fate, altruistically sacrificing his life for the sake of the crew. This was what damaged normal cells did. Like Spock, the sacrifice was made for the sake of the many because that was the right thing to do. However, when it was a cancer cell, they didn't die like they were supposed to for the sake of the many. They grew out of control, driven by selfish means and their own sets of signals to remain alive. Most importantly, cancer cells shut off the death pathway. Figuring out how cancer cells cheated death by turning off the default cell death pathway and how to turn it back on was a goal in cancer research. I liked the simplified definition of life and death. It made studying why cancer cells wouldn't die an intriguing question that drove my research project in graduate school.

I bonded with my graduate death project. I'd had headaches that came out of nowhere since I was thirteen years old. A lifetime of anger had built over pain I was unable to predict or manage, much less control. I was consumed with the mechanisms of how cells died and how I could convince cancer cells to do so. I especially enjoyed killing them because this gave me an outlet for the anger, in a good way. I grew cancer cells and treated them with different drugs to see which ones would turn on the death pathway. Some cancer drugs worked but in other cases, like when the cancers cells were those that represented late-stage or metastatic cancer, the drugs didn't kill them any longer. That was where the challenge began to figure out why that was. I worked with a prostate cancer cell culture model. In the early stage of the disease, the cells could be convinced to commit suicide when treated with cancer drugs but later on, like when the cancer progressed, the cells refused to respond to the drugs. The cells in culture acted like advanced stage prostate cancer and wouldn't turn on the death pathway no matter what I treated them with. It was this critical turning point in cancer cells where I spent most of my graduate work trying to find out how cancer cells sneak past the death pathway. My goal was to get them back on the road to death. By the end of my first year, I'd earned the nickname, Queen of Death, and I was proud of that. It wasn't just because I killed cells and apoptosis was becoming my area of expertise. It was because I felt like I had some control.

Lounging in the armchair on the twelfth floor looking out the bay window of the Research Center, I waited as the 36 hour timed treatment point in the experiment crept near. It was Saturday night, and other than the lights on and hum of incubators in my lab, the twelfth floor was dark and silent. It was an unseasonably warm late September. A high pressure system had settled in over the Midwest pushing temperatures up into the high 90's, sweltering hot for the end of summer. This caused an unusually high pollen bloom and triggered a headache.

I had the experiment set up to incubate at time points over the weekend. I ran a lot of my experiments that way, so they wouldn't interfere with courses, journal club, seminars and the other, usual demands of a graduate student. The timed intervals had to be stopped and processed at 12, 24, and 36 hours. I'd started the experiment on Friday and planned for a long weekend.

My head was pounding, but it was only a few more hours until the last time point was done, then I could wrap up the experiment and go home. I rubbed my eyes and massaged my forehead then stood to stretch before I wandered down the hallway to the lab. My desk was situated between the cell culture room and main lab, in a pass-through hallway designated as clean space. A mini-fridge with a shelf above it that held a coffee pot served as a partition wall, providing a wedge of privacy between my desk and the lab.

I paused for a moment at the shelf and thought about brewing a pot of coffee, then changed my mind as I sunk into my chair and reached under the desk for the small, square pillow I kept tucked away for these late nights. I pushed the chair back to prop my feet up and placed the pillow under my head. Maybe I could grab a quick nap while the last few hours of the experiment passed. It wouldn't be the first time I'd done that. Dr. K. never visited the pass through hallway even though his office was only a few steps away around the corner in front of the main lab. If I needed anything from him, it was up to me to chase him down, which was the way I liked it. The cramped six by six foot open hallway desk space became my home away from home. I was secure in my corner. It was a place I could go to hide but still work when the headaches came. The best part was that no one knew I had them. After five years and four peer reviewed papers published, graduate school was behind me.

My dream job ended with a realization that the headaches limited what I'd be capable. I hung up the phone and jumped from the chair, almost knocking it over as I stood up to the window to look south. I could barely contain the excitement. Dr. F. called and wanted to interview me for the position. I was headed to Miami in a week. I was done with my graduate studies, and had already graduated. I'd applied to several labs for research positions and post docs, but this was my top choice. Located on a sixteen acre beachfront campus, the Rosenstiel Research lab worked in marine field research.

They needed a molecular biologist to help design detection systems, and I was their candidate.

I targeted my applications to the coasts, but I had a special interest in Florida. I'd been gone from home nearly twenty years, and the desire to return was overwhelming. I longed for the sun, ocean and wet sand on my bare feet. I'd been up north for so long I'd forgotten what the waves pushing against the shore looked like. I wanted this bad. I could already taste the salt and hear the sound of ocean waves splashing in my mind. I rehearsed my presentation for the interview dozens of times to make sure it was perfect and read up on the research ongoing at the Rosenstiel Research campus. I was going to make sure I hit a home run on this interview. I knew my own work well but spent a few hours reading papers on marine field research then put together a few extra slides to make sure I had some ideas ready to talk over how I would contribute to this new position. In these interviews, the candidate arrived and gave a seminar to present their work to the department and then the floor opened to questions. This was a way to demonstrate ones character, personality and level of intellectual capability. The day after was for a tour of the lab and facilities to get a feel for the work environment. There was plenty of time in-between for interaction with lab members, other post-doctoral colleagues and most importantly, Dr. F. who would serve as my new mentor.

I packed my best suit along with some shorts, sandals and T-shirt for the trip as Dr. F. recommended when we spoke on the phone. We had a special tour to take as part of the interview. The flight was scheduled to leave early on Sunday. I'd take a shuttle to the hotel then meet Dr. F. and some of the lab members for an informal dinner later that night. I went to bed early Saturday before the trip, but couldn't sleep because the excitement kept me awake. I tossed and turned in anticipation and was little worried, too, because the air pressure changes I'd go through during the flight might spur a headache. That had happened to me before when I'd flown. I packed a full box of BC powders and hoped for the best.

I stepped out of the airport terminal to find a shuttle. The warmth began to sink in as I decompressed from the too cold, air conditioned flight and long layover in Atlanta. I squinted against the bright, Florida sun then reached into my bag for the sunglasses I'd brought along. As I slid them on my face, I felt the all too familiar tingling on the right side of my head. I shrugged it off, but in the pit of my stomach, worry grew because I knew what it was. I had a few hours before time to meet Dr. F. and the lab crew for dinner. Once I found a shuttle and got checked into the hotel, I could take a BC, splash cool water on my face to freshen up and rest for a while.

"I'll be right down," I said as my heart raced in excited anticipation hanging up the hotel phone. It was Dr. F. He was waiting downstairs with the group from the lab. I jumped from the bed and tossed the wet washcloth I was using to cool my forehead into the sink. The tingling that had started earlier had advanced to a full-on headache. I was trying to meditate the pain to manageable and must have dozed off briefly. I straightened my hair and checked to make sure my clothes had not become too disheveled while I rested then grabbed my bag and hurried down to the lobby.

A sticky breeze filtered between the high rise hotels in downtown Miami as we walked. The smell of salt from the Atlantic Ocean and ethnic foods simmering drifted out from the kitchens of specialty restaurants. Art deco hues exploded and changed with each venue as we passed storefronts. People of all countries and origins hurried on their way around us. Some were dressed casually and others, in formal suits. I wanted Miami to become my home. If all went well during this multiple days' interview it could but with every step, it felt like a knife stabbed through the front of my head, and my stomach churned as acid boiled. We carried on our polite conversation, and I smiled as we arrived at the café and sat at an outdoor table.

*How will I eat without throwing up?* I thought as the waiter delivered plates of food to the table adjoining ours, and the invading aromas drifted over. I sipped on a glass of ice water to clear my palate of the smell as we began talking about the different projects Dr. F. had going on in his lab. The cold water helped to settle the uneasiness in my stomach. By the time it was our tables turn to order, I was feeling confident and picked out one of my favorites from the menu, a chicken Caesar salad. I continued to sip on the ice water. Drinking cold water was helpful when I had headaches but only a little. What I wanted to do was unfold my politely folded napkin, dunk it in the cold water and tie it around my head like a bandana. That would be more helpful than drinking it, but that would blow my cover.

Our food arrived quickly. My stomach turned as the salad landed in front of me. I let out slow and steady breaths between tiny bites of Romaine lettuce with shards of parmesan cheese embedded in drippings of Caesar dressing. Normally one of my favorite salads, it was torture to eat when my head hurt. Dr. F. and the lab crew dug in to eat quickly. They were too busy to notice my aversion to the food until Dr. F. looked over.

"It was a long flight, and I grabbed something during the layover in Atlanta," I responded in an effort to explain why most of my salad was untouched. Dr. F. finished his meal and then folded his napkin and placed it on the table. The waiter arrived to collect our plates. He took Dr. F.'s empty plate first and then reached over for mine.

"Would you like this boxed?" The waiter offered as he swung around to the other side of the table to see if the others were done. I nodded yes. I hadn't eaten much. When the headache reached this intensity, it was too risky to eat. My stomach was already tight with nervousness, and now the pain was making it churn. The sun went down, and a breeze picked up. My head felt a little better with the dimmed light as we continued to dig further into details of the project. I needed to get as much information as I could about what I'd be doing for the position.

"Can we tweak the French press underwater?" Dr. F. asked, his eyebrows raised and hands lifted up to shoulder height looking over the table for my response. That sparked excitement and I forgot about the headache long enough to discuss how we might get together and do it. The French pressure cell press, or French press for short, was a method we used to bust open cells. It was a mechanical approach to tear into a cell using physical force where a cell was pushed through an opening smaller than its size. The result was that the cell was ripped apart, and its contents spilled out. The cell innards squished out of the French press landed on a detector which identified what kinds of marine microorganisms were present. What we wanted to do was design one of these on a detection system and place it five miles off the coast of Miami and twenty feet underwater in the Atlantic Ocean. The project had paramount challenges and needed a team of experts to make it all come together. A molecular biologist, who knew something about killing cells in unusual ways, was motivated and willing to dive in the water to make it work and wanted to live in South Florida were all a good start. It had my name written all over it.

We ended the evening with a plan for Dr. F. to pick me up from the hotel first thing in the morning to drive to the Rosenstiel Research campus. There was a tight timeline in place for the next day, so I'd grab breakfast at the hotel since the presentation was scheduled for 9am. Walking back to the hotel with the group, I was exhausted and relieved but felt positive about the impression I'd made despite the pounding headache. *I can do this*, I thought.

Back in my room, I abandoned the chicken Caesar salad leftovers in the to-go box on the desk and grabbed for a packet of BC. The powdery dust slid onto my tongue, and I swallowed it down with a room temperature cup of water from the bathroom sink. I undressed, climbed in the shower and let the steam soak into my body until I was numb then fell into bed with hopes that the headache would be over by next morning. I needed to be rested and fresh for the next day.

The headache wouldn't let me find a comfortable position for a moment of sleep. Between excitement for the coming day and continued pounding in my head, I was awake all night. By morning, I was able to eat only a few bites from the hotel breakfast bar to wash down another BC. I didn't want to take it on an empty stomach and risk getting sick on such an important day. I was waiting in the hotel lobby when Dr. F. pulled in the roundabout.

"You have all of your stuff for the day?" Dr. F. asked as I jumped in the passenger seat and slid my bag on the floor in front of my feet. I confirmed, and we picked up on the conversation from the night before on the French press. Dr. F. cracked the window to let in some fresh air, and a rush of early morning warm humidity filtered in. I smelled the Atlantic Ocean before I saw it. As we turned from US1 onto the causeway leading out to Virginia Key, I saw the morning sunrise flickering on the wave crests. It made me forget about the headache as we finished the drive to the research campus.

Department faculty filtered in. A few stopped to chat with Dr. F. who greeted them in the doorway as I checked the computer and loaded the file onto the desktop. I was calm and well prepared as the lights lowered, but my head throbbed and stomach tightened into a knot. I'd given dozens of presentations to important audiences before. I knew how to focus past the nervousness, but this was different. I raised my chin, pulled my shoulders back and began the presentation with a firm voice, thanking the Rosenstiel Research faculty for their gracious invitation and began with an overview. I explained how I treated cells with different toxins, bursts them open, took out their DNA and ran analyses. Main points were met with nods of approval as I made eye contact with audience members. Across my forehead, folds of pain from the headache were hidden, etched under the guise of intensity for my work.

Fifty minutes passed quickly. I concluded the presentation, thanked the department again for the hospitable invitation and asked the audience for questions. A hearty applause was followed by rounds of detailed queries about my techniques and how I'd adapt them. I planned for that. I had slides ready and spent the next ten minutes proposing how I would construct a hypothetical model to tweak the French press to detect microbe DNA underwater. I glanced over to see Dr. F. gleaming with satisfaction. He was pleased. A last round of applause concluded, and the audience headed towards the exits. I breathed a sigh of relief as the lights were turned back on. Adrenalin from the presentation had worn off, and the headache intensified. There were no breaks scheduled into the day. I wouldn't be going back to the hotel where I could take a BC, splash water on my face and rest. The plan was for me to slip into the ladies room and change into my shorts, T-shirt and sandals for the tour, but what I really needed was an extended break to hide in the dark, lay a cold washcloth on my forehead to try and get the headache under control. There was no time for that. This was the day when everything happened.

"There's pastries left if you want to grab one," Dr. F. said, tilting his head to gesture down at the rejected leftovers on the table as he refilled his coffee mug with tepid brew.

"No, I'm good," I replied as I closed out the presentation file, deleted it from the desktop and clicked through the shutdown sequence for the computer. The thought of a stale sticky bun made my stomach turn despite the fact that I was starving. The risk of getting sick was too real to ruin the interview and plans for the day.

I felt and looked more like one of the lab crew once I changed into my casual clothes except that my legs hung pasty northern white from the black, dress shorts I'd brought to wear for the tour. Dr. F. was wearing khaki shorts, a button down shirt untucked and Top Sider boat shoes. Most everyone we passed in the halls on the way over to start the research lab tour wore shorts and sandals despite the general lab safety rules of long pants and closed toed shoes. That was how we dressed back home where I worked, but this research facility was nothing like where I came from.

I dropped off my tightly folded suit and shoes stuffed into the gym bag in Dr. F.'s office then we stopped, and I was introduced to the department secretary. She'd take care of my processing paperwork if an offer was made, and I got the position. We continued on towards the wing where the research lab was located passing by a continual row of floor-length windows that looked out onto white sand beaches. Virginia Key was located due north of Key Biscayne accessed via a causeway from mainland Miami. The Rosenstiel Research Campus shared the barrier island with a marine aquarium, the fisheries service and NOAA all nestled on the southwestern nub of the island.

Dr. F.'s lab was the last one on the first floor, tucked in the corner of the research building. He swung the door open, and we entered into the wet lab greeted by a warm hint of brine in the air. Two sets of long, black-top benches were arranged parallel to floor length windows, similar to those we had just walked past through the main corridor. Dr. F. disappeared through an opening towards the back of the lab. I moved toward the windows, interested in a pier I could see far off in the distance.

"You can sit outside or walk down to the dock," Dr. F. said as he returned. "Some of the crew sits outside at the tables to have their lunches," he continued, pointing to a sidewalk that led to a set of metal picnic tables arranged along its path. "And, that's our research vessel docked over there," Dr. F. explained, as he lifted one hand to form a visor to shield his eyes from the sun cresting above the horizon and pointed into the distance towards the pier with his other hand. "Let's take a look at the lab then we'll get everyone together and head over," he finished and turned, lowering his hand-visor just as a ray of sunlight caught the anticipation in his eyes.

The last part of the tour was a trip out on the research vessel. We were headed five miles off the coast of Miami to see where we planned to place the microbe DNA detectors-- the ones I would invent. After we toured the main lab and I saw the saltwater tanks setup to immerse test detectors in the room adjacent to the wet lab, and the modern molecular biology lab, I didn't need any more convincing. I felt like I was ready to get started even though my head throbbed as I tried to take in all the details of where everything was.

"It's a beautiful day, don't you think?" Dr. F.'s voice resonated as we stood on the dock waiting for the lab crew to finish gathering.

*My God, It was!* I thought in agreement. I looked up at Dr. F. and nodded. This was the most fantastic adventure I'd be undertaking in the last twenty years had it not been for the excruciating pain in my head. I took in a deep breath and smiled as I raised my head up towards the boat. The thick, sea air expanded in my lungs and brought a moment of relief until exhale left the pain building. Under the careful disguise of sunglasses, the sinking under my eyes was hidden. Being out in the sun when these headaches struck was the worst.

"You don't get seasick do you?" Dr. F. asked as he sprung over the gap between the pier and the vessel then offered his hand to help me board. I shook my head, no, as I grabbed for the railing and hopped on deck. The sudden move and slight rocking of the vessel made my legs unsteady. I had eaten only a few bites of a bagel early that morning, more than six hours previously. With the pounding headache, intense sun and dropping blood sugar, I stumbled and nearly fell. I caught myself on the railing at the last minute.

"You OK?" Dr. F. cried out in a panic as he jumped towards me, faster than I would have imagined capable for a man his age, as he reached out and tried to help.

"It's OK. I mean… I'm OK," I correct myself as I better steadied against the sidewall. I hadn't been on a vessel in the ocean since I was in my teens. I wasn't prepared for the subtle rocking motion, the bright sunlight or the unexpected headache that was ruining my dream job interview.

It was cooler as we distanced the vessel from the coast. The lab crew was at home on the boat and took their comfortable positions under the canopy. It was just a trip to out to work for them but not that day. We'd spend it visiting the locations where the sensors were placed and enjoy the ocean. It was all part of the interview.

"We dive down to the buoys and place the detectors. You'll get your divers certification once you're setup and ready to go," Dr. F. explained as we surveyed a printed map that plotted the different locations of each target buoy. I looked at the map, but the pain in my head was pushing against my eyes, and I couldn't focus to see the fine details. I shook my head and agreed anyway, following along as Dr. F. pointed, outlined and explained the marks, as if we were already in our diving gear swimming along underwater visiting each detector. It made me dizzy, and a haze started to form around the outline of his hand, the map and the table. Then, the nausea set in.

I turned and left the shade of the canopy to stand starboard, with the sun behind my back, pretending to search for the distant buoys I'd studied moments before on the printed map. I closed my eyes and drifted with the waves in a moment of desperate meditation. My thoughts wandered as my hands tightened to a white-knuckled grip on the aluminum railing. I was squeezing so hard, it seemed my palms might push dents into them. I felt the vessels movement as waves of nausea welled up, beads of sweat poured across my cheeks, and I fought to hold back.

"Are you OK?" Dr. F. raised his voice to ask as he approached placing his hand on my shoulder with a reassuring pat. "Maybe you're having a case of seasickness?" he continued.

"No, no, I'm not seasick…it's …," my voice trailed. "This reminds me of my father when we used to go out in our boat years ago," I insisted weakly as efforts to hide the nausea and pain continued to break down. Being out there did remind me of the last time I spent with my dad, but the pain was out of control. We were on a boat, miles off the coast, and I had nowhere to hide this headache. As I loosened my grip from the bow railing to head back under the canopy, my legs gave out, and I stumbled. This time, Dr. F. caught my fall.

"It feels a little warm out today. Let's get a bottle of cold water and sit under the canopy," Dr. F. suspiciously reassured as he half carried, half led me back to the shade as the lab crew watched, wide-eyed and disappointed.

The fantasy ended late in the afternoon. We docked as the sun began to perch over the tops of high rises across downtown Miami. Dr. F. drove me to the hotel as my flight was scheduled to leave early the next morning. I was relieved to be out of the sun and back inside the comforts of the hotel room. I grabbed a washcloth, ran some cold water over it and then laid it across my forehead. I collapsed on the bed and dozed for a while. It was dark when I woke. I needed to catch the first shuttle out in the morning, and my clothes weren't packed. I called down to the lobby to schedule my shuttle and order room service, but the restaurant was already closed for the day. I hung up the phone and rolled out of bed. My stomach knotted as I stood. It had been two days since I'd had a full meal, and I was starving. I looked over to the chicken Caesar salad to-go box still sitting on the desk. Room cleaning must have left it. *Thank God*, I thought as my mouth watered in anticipation as I reached over and popped it open. The smell of spoiled parmesan and rancid oil from the dressing wafted out of the box and clung to my face. The Romaine lettuce was no longer recognizable. It was wilted pools of slime with chunks of fuzzy chicken embedded. I slammed the container closed, my appetite gone, and tossed it in the trash.

The letter arrived two weeks after I got home from the interview. They thanked me for taking the time to fly out to give a seminar. They found my research fascinating. They appreciated my interest and enthusiasm in the job, but they didn't offer me the position. I wasn't invited to join the research group. There would be no French press detectors invented in the lab, no breaks midday walking along Virginia Key beach to gather my thoughts for the next experiment and no dives off the coast to place detectors on buoys.

The headache had won.

I knew when Dr. F. dropped me off at the hotel that evening in Miami it was over. I couldn't be the reason a mission to place detectors was put off because of a random headache. They made me sick enough that I wouldn't be capable of contributing. Dr. F. didn't know that because I didn't tell him. If I told anyone, I wouldn't have received an interview in the first place. Even though I did everything I could to hide the headaches, I discovered what my limits with them were.

It's Just a Headache

\*\*\*

I turned off the AC and hit the button to lower the window. It was nearing 90 degrees outside, and I'd moved less than two blocks in the last ten minutes. I would have taken an alternate route if I'd known it was like this. Maybe there was an accident holding up traffic, but I couldn't see past the line of vehicles ahead. It was only a twelve mile drive, and everyone used the two lane highway leading out of the industrial park triangle. I'd started the new position two weeks ago, and was still getting accustomed to the commute. It was summer in Eastern North Carolina, and I looked forward to the end of the day and a dip in the pool, especially today. It was usually an hour drive but today would be much longer at this rate. I dialed home again but no one answered.

The sun was low on the horizon when I pulled in at home. I saw the Toyota parked in the driveway and lights on inside the house through the living room windows. As I walked around to enter the house from the back door that led into the kitchen, the cobblestone steps were flooded, but it hadn't rained that day. Over the deck and next to the ladder leading into the pool, inflated rafts, a beach ball, wet towels and empty soda bottles were strewn.

"Mom, where have you been? The pool's leaking, and we're hungry," my daughter said in an anxious voice as I wiped the water off my shoes on the entry door mat then dropped my briefcase on the floor as the back door closed behind me and I reached up to flipped on the outdoor light.

I'd secured a research position with the US Government in North Carolina. It was a huge step up after only a year as a post-doctoral fellow at Boystown National Research Hospital. I'd traveled out ahead of time to house shop and chose a two story, three bedrooms, and three bathroom colonial style with a pool nestled in a small town a few miles outside of the city. I knew the kids would love the privacy of their own bathroom, and we needed more space. The townhouse we were leaving behind in Nebraska was cramped. I wanted make sure we had a smooth transition to our new home. I was moving the kids over a thousand miles across the country away from their friends, extended family and during their impressionable teen years.

We arrived to our new home in July, over a month before the kids would begin school and two weeks prior to my start date at the new job. The usual chaos ensued getting settled as I rushed to get the house setup and functional. Our belongings had made it in one piece including the kid's car trailered inside a special moving truck. They were excited they'd be off on their own to check out the town. The pool was a centerpiece. Leaving other, more pressing home agenda undone, we filled it, added the chemicals and tested to make sure the water was in proper equilibrium. The kids wasted no time making friends as teen pool parties started the moment the girls put their bikinis on and jumped in. The first two weeks flew by in the harried pace of getting settled. I had to get to work. I left the kids to their pool, the car to explore the town and a kitchen full of snacks to share with their new friends. But like any honeymoon, everything was great at first then the cracks started to show in the morning sunlight.

I'd put in a special request at work for time off, so the girls and I could head over to the Department of Motor Vehicles. The 30-day limit on our driver's licenses was about to expire, and we needed to change them over. I figured if we arrived early, we'd beat the crowd. The line stretched out the door at 7:45am, fifteen minutes before the DMV was scheduled to open. The girls had got out of bed before 5am to take showers, style their hair and put on makeup. They were picture-perfect for the new driver's license photos. Their patience after the hour and a half wait ended abruptly when the official took their Nebraska provisional licenses and informed them they would be able to drive only to and from school or work. North Carolina provisional driver's licenses for teens under the age of 18 were restrictive.

"You have the pool, once it gets repaired, and your new friends to hang out with until school starts," I reassured the girls in an effort to ease the loss of their driving privileges as I dropped them off at home on my way back to work. I had to get back to the lab. I was still in the first month of the new position and needed to show that I was dependable. My days at the lab were growing longer as I transitioned, and the project picked up steam, but the problems kept coming up at home. Getting settled was a little harder and more expensive than I had planned.


My thumb sunk into the soft dough as I reached for the pizza in the freezer. If it hadn't been for the cardboard support underneath and vacuum sealed plastic wrapper, the pizza would have folded in half when I lifted it. Thinking that the problem may have been limited to something wrong with only the freezer, I opened the refrigerator below to see the light was on, but my hand felt room temperature against the side walls, and the milk was warm. The refrigerator was full. I'd made a double cart load trip to the grocery store and stocked it to the brim two days before. The freezer was crammed with easy-to-make frozen goodies like pizzas, microwave sandwiches and ice cream bars which were the kinds of foods the kids liked and made for quick dinners since I was arriving home closer to 6:30 to 7pm from work most evenings. It was already too late to get someone out to look at the refrigerator to see what was wrong and if it could be repaired. I baked the soggy pizza for dinner, tossed the mushy ice cream bars in the trash and packed the one Igloo cooler we had with the remaining salvaged food and covered it with a bag of ice I picked up after dinner from the only open gas station in town. Three days later and a new bag of ice added each day to the cooler I picked up on my way home from work; the repair man let me know that buying a new refrigerator was the better option than trying to fix the old one. Two more days, $900 plus a delivery charge on my credit card, the old refrigerator was wheeled away, and the new one sat empty, ice cold and ready to be filled again.

The pool repairman showed up at the house while I was at work. I knew the liner was leaking, and I'd probably need a new one, but when the call came to my desk that the pump also had some mechanical problem, and the total doubled, I pulled out the credit card again. I was getting a deal on the labor, or so the technician said, since he was already there and could fix the problem with the pump while he emptied the pool and changed out the old liner for a new one. With the girls stuck at home without driving privileges and school another month away, at least the pool would be up and running again, I rationalized to myself, as I read off the numbers to my credit card over the phone.

"It's how much?" I questioned pulling the debit card back a second before the pharmacy technician grabbed it out of my hand.

"That will be $167, please," she repeated, loudly, embarrassing me and irritated I was holding up the line.

"Can you check that total? I have insurance for my prescriptions," I asked quietly and politely, my face burning red in embarrassment. She grimaced and looked over my head at the line behind me then turned and disappeared back into the pharmacy. I'd already spent over $250 on my daughters' prescriptions that month. They weren't available in generic. I was left with no options for less expensive refills to keep her asthma under control. My triptans didn't cost this much to refill back in Nebraska. I'd have to find out why the sudden increase.

"Your copay is $187 for the three injections. We'll need to get an approval for the three tablets. Your copay on those is $89,"the technician reported as she returned to the counter holding the bag with my prescriptions close to her but out of my reach in one hand and then waved her fingers in a gesture for payment in the other. A quick addition in my head came to over $250 for my prescriptions. Together, that meant between my daughter and I, this was going to run close to $600 every month. I slid the debit card back into my wallet and flipped out the credit card to pay, as I'd been doing a lot of lately. I was getting six doses of medicine to treat over fifteen headaches a month. That was not going to work. The active prescription I'd brought from Nebraska was about to expire, and I needed to find a local doctor within the new insurance network before the pharmacy cut me off from the few doses of triptans they were giving me. I took the kids in first and found replacement doctors for them but put mine off until the pharmacist refused to fill any more of my refills. Then, I went in search of a triptan drug dealer.

The office was close to my work, so I could squeeze in midafternoon, lunch hour appointments because I didn't want to take paid time off to go. I showed up for the first appointment early, as the receptionist said I should in order to complete the new patient information forms. The fingerprint smudged glass entry doors opened into the waiting room where about a half-dozen people sat. The room was stale, as if the air conditioning wasn't working. An oversized banana leaf blade-shaped ceiling fan spun slowly but did little to cool the area. I nodded a half smile to the waiting patients as I walked past them and checked in with the receptionist. She handed me a clipboard with a stapled stack of pages attached and instructed that I should complete all of them thoroughly. I took the clipboard with the paperwork to a seat and started on the process of filling them out. Seven pages later and after I dug out my address book (the little back one from the bottom of my purse) to find names, addresses and numbers of previous doctors and emergency contacts, I finished the stack of forms then returned them to the check in counter. I noticed as I turned to head towards my seat that no one had been called back since I'd arrived.

Forty-five minutes later, my name was called to disappear behind the door. I noticed right away how much cooler it was in the patient prep area than in the waiting room. I was weighed, my blood pressure was checked and then I was escorted to a patient exam room by the nurse to wait some more. At least it was cooler as I sat in the exam room reading magazines another thirty minutes before the doctor arrived. An obese woman in her mid-40's entered dressed in a long floral patterned skirt and white, quarter sleeve collared blouse. I could have easily mistaken her for one of the waiting room patients because she wasn't wearing a white doctor's coat. Visibly sweating, I could hear her labored breathing. I greeted the doctor appropriately as she returned an acknowledgement in kind. She sat on the stool and began her review of the papers attached to a clipboard she had carried in, presumably the new patient information forms I had completed out in the lobby.

"Your insurance is Blue Cross, and you're here for headaches?" The doctor asked as she briefly looked up at me. I shook my head and confirmed as she scribbled some notes on the top page of my forms. After a brief peek at the last page in the stack, she reached over and grabbed onto the counter to help hoist up her mass then rose from the stool and moved towards the door. "Check with the receptionist about what pharmacy to send the prescriptions and I'll see you again in six months," the doctor's voice labored as she turned the handle. I interrupted as she began to leave and asked how many doses of the triptans she had prescribed. "Your insurance will pay part of one set of injections and one set of tablets a month," she replied as the door closed behind her.

It wasn't enough. That was nine doses of medicine. There were plenty of days when I needed to take more than one dose to get a headache under control, but the doctor didn't stay in the room long enough, didn't ask me any relevant medical questions and didn't even look at me for more than a few seconds much less perform a physical examination. I'd already been gone from work more than two hours for what I had planned on a one hour lunch break appointment. I grabbed my purse and hurried to the receptionist's desk down the hall to setup the pharmacy, passing the doctor struggling to walk to the next patient two exam rooms down from mine. I nodded, politely at the doctor as I squeezed by.

I hurried back to work hoping my boss hadn't noticed how long I'd been gone. I thought I could sneak in by taking a long walk and looping around the hallway to slip in through the lab via a door that opened discreetly into my office. This route wouldn't pass my bosses office through the front hallway. I popped in the back door to find my boss standing there waiting to go over some plans for the next weeks' experiments. I knew he'd been there a while when he glanced down at his watch as I settled into my chair and slid my purse under the desk. The prescriptions were hanging out of the top, and I didn't want him to see them. He didn't ask where I'd been for so long, and I was glad because I didn't want to share that information with him.

The next Monday morning, I had to drop everything and leave work suddenly. Everything had been going smoothly at home for a while and a sense of order had set in once school started. Sleeping in late, lounging around the pool and staying up half the night watching TV was replaced with a regular routine. Though the girls didn't appear completely adjusted to the new school, they seemed happy about being able to drive their car to get there. I was already gone that morning since I left daily at 6am to avoid rush hour traffic. I was wrapping up an early morning lab meeting when I got the call. The Toyota wouldn't start, and the girls needed a ride to school. I didn't say anything to my boss. I grabbed my keys and purse and ran out the door. I could make it a quick trip there and back, and maybe he wouldn't notice. Thinking my boss would be headed back to his office after our morning meeting, I slipped out the back door of my lab. I was headed for the loop towards the exit when I ran into him reading over his notes from our morning meeting. My keys and purse in hand, I looked up at him with a nervous smile and let him know I'd be right back. I rushed home, the girls jumped in, and I drove them to school but didn't have time to check the car until that evening. The engine did nothing when the key turned, so I called the only repair shop in town the next day and made arrangements for them to have the car towed in.

A tow truck backed into the driveway the following Saturday morning. The driver got out and walked around to the side of the Toyota and bent down to size up the job. He reached under to feel for something then wiped both hands down the front of his pants as he stood. Black skid marks from his mid-thigh to the end of his shirt tail suggested he'd done a few jobs. I put on my shoes and headed out the front door of the house. As I got closer, the faint efforts of an evergreen Little Tree air freshener failed to hide the overflowing ash tray inside the cab of the tow truck. The driver removed straps from the back and began securing them to the front tires.

"I can drop the keys off if you want," the driver said as he pushed back on the handle engaging the hydraulic lift raising the front of the car. A creaking sound started as it rose, and pieces of rust fell onto the driveway. Spots of oil and a sizeable pool of a reddish-colored liquid were visible under the engine on the concrete. I thought for a minute, no, I shouldn't give a stranger the keys and then decided it would save an hour or more and anyway, it's a small town- - where else would he take an old Toyota that doesn't start other than the only repair shop in town. I handed him the keys, a check and watched as the car bounced behind the tow truck as he carted it out of the driveway, down the street and turned. The school bus stop was at the corner where he turned. The girls would have to walk there to catch the bus in the mornings for a while. I couldn't be late for work as some long days were coming up.

"You do the heads, and I'll do the brains," the technician instructed as we pushed the cart stacked with cages clear of the doorway. I turned and checked the handle to make sure the door locked behind us. Even though there was no bedding in the fresh cages, the smell of urine soaked pine and feces lingered as we pushed the cart down the access hall towards the cell culture prep facility. We didn't waste prepped cages or those with a fresh layer of bedding, a water bottle and a tray of feed pellets. These subjects didn't need all that. We pulled the cart into the room, and I pushed it over to the side where I'd be working then reached up to flip on the light. The subjects scurried to find a dark corner at the sudden intrusion. Nocturnal by nature, they knew to run from light to try and find a place to hide in the dark even though they were less than two weeks old.

The technician and I began our preparations for the procedure starting with our PPE. She poked her head into the opening of an apron and as it hung loose around her neck, pulled the sides wide open to find the tie strings to secure them behind her. Tugging hard on the breast cover, she was careful to make sure it was pulled up far enough to protect her shirt collar, placed a mesh cap over her hair then slid the first pair of gloves on her hands. I followed suit and donned my PPE then we both got started on setting up our work areas. My table was to the left of the sterile cell culture hood where I laid out a bench diaper, extra pairs of gloves and the scissors. In the back corner of the table, I placed a one liter sized tub lined with a red biohazard plastic bag and to my right, a squirt bottle filled with disinfectant. The cart stacked with cages was parked sideways, behind me for easy access. Inside the cell culture hood, the technician setup a ring stand with a large 10x magnifying glass, sterile scalpels, tweezers and extra-long pins lay to her left. Petri dishes prefilled with growth media were pushed to the far right and awaited seeding of cortical cells.

"Are you ready?" I asked the technician as I sprayed my gloved hands with disinfectant and then sat the bottle down on the cart next to the cages within easy reach.

"Let's get started, "she replied, letting out a long breath as she pulled the second set of gloves over the first making sure they pinched closed the ends of her sleeves. I looked over into the first cage. They were a scrawny group that day. Small subjects meant small brains, but they were all at least 10-days and some were 2-weeks old. We couldn't let them get any older else, the cells wouldn't work right for the experiment. It was now or never. They were huddled together in pink blobs trying to stay warm. We'd placed seven to eight per cage, which was about two litters in each, so they could until it was time. They needed to remain alive. Any dead ones or runts would be unusable. It was my turn to do the heads, and part of that was I had to separate out the dead and decide which ones might be runts. The trip from the animal facility to cell culture prep was traumatizing, and it was not unusual for one or two to die. I'd find the dead lump of a carcass sucked up and stuck in the huddles. The runts were more of a subjective call. I pushed those aside until last.

The technician glared up at me anxious for the first delivery. I grabbed the disinfectant and gave my hands another quick spray then pried the first one from the pack. The 10-day old mouse was about the size of my thumb. Careful to grip the tiny pup by its mostly furless, loose skin, I felt the packs warmth still radiating through the tiny animal as I separated it from the group. Perhaps thinking its mother had come to save it, the pup's limbs grasped around my finger, claws not yet developed enough to pierce through the thick, double layers of latex. Holding the pup in my left hand, I turned it over on its back, stretched and pinched its tail with my pinky and secured the abdomen with my ring and middle finger. With my index finger and thumb, I formed a noose around the shoulders, careful to ensure the front limbs were pinned under my thumb. And in my right hand, I grabbed the scissors and approached from underneath then squeezed to tighten the noose at the last moment, so the neck stretched and extended. The cut was hard, fast and decapitation was complete. In my left hand, I held the headless body of the pup, and on the bench diaper, the head rested.

I sat the scissors aside then pinched hold of the nearly weightless head by the severed edge of its neck and passed it over to the technician to dissect the cortical cells from the brain under the confines of the culture hood. She misted the severed head, using her bottle of disinfectant, until it dripped wet with a tinge of pinkish-red blood then mounted it face down with the long, sterile pins under the magnifying glass. Tweezers in one hand and a scalpel in the other, she started the dissection. The 10-day old mouse pup skull was not hardened bone but more like peeling the skin of a peach to find a fingernail covered the surface of the brain. Once the sets of cuts were made, the delicate folds of baby skin were pushed back, and the scalpel was used to gently carve then clip away the thin layer of skull to reveal the brain. A new set of sterile tweezers and scalpel was used to dissect down to the cortex which was where the cells we wanted were located. There were only a few of them there.

I felt the pups' cold, headless body in my left hand continue to convulse. The struggle had started when I tightened my fist around it. Seconds before the scissors signaled the exit of its head, the pup knew something was wrong and in a panic, made a last ditch effort to escape. Even after the head left, the front and back legs jerked in sync as if the pup was trying to run away but was getting nowhere. When the spinal cord was severed, the final signal sent from the brain to the motor neurons left the pup convulsing using energy it had stored in its muscle cells.

I dropped the pup's body into the one liter biohazard container. The jerking front and back legs crunched rhythmically against the stiff red plastic liner. Crunch…crunch…crunch…crunch the sound followed me as I turned back toward the cell culture hood to wait the ten to fifteen minutes it would take for the technician to finish off the first brain. They had to be fresh. I checked to see if she was ready before I grabbed another pup to snip off its head. Crunch….crunch….crunch….the convulsing jerks slowed in the biohazard container behind me as I watched the technician scoop out the tiny group of cells from the cortex and place them into the waiting Petri dish. She pulled out the long, mounting pins and handed me what was left of the mangled head to dispose of it.

Crunch......crunch......movement ceased as I dropped the head into the bucket with the rest of its body.

Some headless bodies convulsed only briefly. Others continued on five or more minutes though the flexing limbs would slow as time went on until they stopped completely. The rare ones never did. I second guessed my judgement on those that didn't convulse at all and wondered if they were ill chosen runts that should have been pushed aside and never used in the experiments. We scooped out about a BB-sized amount of the cortical cells from each brain, so it took 20 to 30 mouse pups to make an experiment work. The number we used depended on the size of the average 10-day to 2-week old pup. How large or small a pup was a birth went back to the way the experiment was designed.

Most of what went wrong in a developing brain happened before birth or while the brain finished its development in a young pup. We poisoned the pregnant mothers or took the brain cells from normal pups and poisoned them after they were grown up in Petri dishes. Pregnant mothers were fed, injected or exposed to teratogens or things that influenced the embryonic development of their pups. In those cases, the pups were born smaller than normal. For the Petri dish experiments, we dissected cells from completely normal mouse pup brains then treated the cells with poisons once the cells got settled into the Petri dishes. We wanted to understand what neurotoxins did to the brain both from mother to pup and from the environment to the pup. We measured changes in the cortical brain cells connections to each other, the way they sent signals along their axons or even if they were able to respond to normal stimuli. All of this was done in follow-up experiments, but I was left to wonder if the poisons we dumped in the pregnant mothers feed or into the Petri dishes after normal cells were growing caused pain, like headaches. I sure knew what that felt like but didn't know of any quantitative way to measure it. We didn't have any experiments for that.

One after the other, we processed the healthier-looking mouse pups until all that was left were the few straggling runts. I could take them back to the animal facility, check them into the outgoing room, fill out the form, and they'd be taken care of. But, that meant they would sit alone overnight in the same empty cage, and it had already been close to seven hours since we'd taken them from their mother. They weren't going back to her. If I took them back, the animal husbandry technician would give them a final tour of the gas chamber when he arrived into work the next morning. To save myself a trip and the technician the trouble the next day, I grabbed the scissors, snipped off their heads, dumped them into the biohazard container and finished cleaning my work area with disinfectant.

Back at my desk, I sunk into the chair. The green light flashing on the side of my phone indicated there was a voice message, probably from the auto repair shop. I called voicemail then keyed in my password. I knew the bad news was coming. The Toyota needed a transmission, and there were some other engine problems they wanted to discuss with me. It was best if I stopped by after work so we could go over it, the manager said on my voice mail. It was already close to 5pm, and I needed to take care of some other lab duties before I could leave. I flipped the cover closed then shoved the phone in my purse and tucked it back under the desk. I grabbed the stack of material sheets then headed into the main lab to finish up my other lab duties for the day. I'd wait until tomorrow to call back, since the car would likely get sold for scrap. I wasn't in any hurry to disappoint the girls about the car. Glen had purchased tickets for them to fly home to Nebraska for a long weekend visit. I'd let that excitement overshadow things for the time being and wait to deliver

the likely bad news about the car until after they came
home.

***

"What do you mean they're not coming back?" I asked Glen as he listened on the other end of the phone.

"They don't like it there, they can't drive when they want and they miss their friends here," he replied apologetically. I could hear it in his voice. He was relieved the girls had decided not to board the plane home from their long weekend visit. "It's OK," he continued, pausing for a moment, "they can live with me."

I didn't see this one coming. I paced through the house trying to understand as we talked. Upstairs, their rooms looked like they were off to school, with their beds unmade and clothes strewn about. In the bathroom, used towels hung tossed over the shower curtain rod left to dry. As I returned downstairs, I saw the overfilled basket of dirty clothes in the laundry room and in the kitchen, the new refrigerator waited full of their favorite foods I'd hauled in from the grocery store two days before. None of that mattered now because they weren't coming back home. We finished our conversation to work out the details, and I hung up the phone. A silence I hadn't heard before set in as I continued through the house, suddenly lost in the cleanup I was in before the phone call came about the girls not coming home. Reassessing where I was, I needed to get some clothes sent off, but first I had to get them washed.

I shouldn't have moved them across the country at such an impressionable age. I was gone all the time at the new job, and so many unexpected expenses had come up. It was everything I could do to keep up with the demands at work and by the time I got home, dinner, a few chores and errands left little to no free time to enjoy why we had moved across the country in the first place. I was racking up debt on three credit cards trying to keep up with everything that kept breaking. I couldn't just leave and move back. I was under a contract to remain at least a year in my new job. I had no choice for the time being, and I had a mortgage on a two story home that had only started payments six months before.

The multipack stacks of shipping boxes I picked up from the moving store were cheap, until I crammed them full and they weighed in at the post office. That was when it got expensive. I shipped over a dozen across the country packed with clothes, shoes and whatever the girls asked for out of their bedrooms. That was because I didn't have the time off earned from work to drive their stuff over to them. As the rooms emptied with each box filled and shipped off, the house grew quiet, and I dreaded coming home from work. The times I was home on a day off from work, it was with a headaches I didn't have medicine to treat.

My health insurance in North Carolina wouldn't pay for enough medicine to match the number of headaches I had every month, so I saved the doses of triptans I was allotted for work days only. I spent my sick time, PTO and vacation days at home with headaches I had no medicine to treat. I even made a desperate trip to the doctor's office and begged for free triptan sales rep samples, but the new concept of medication overuse was beginning to take hold.

I waited in the lobby while the nurse disappeared to ask the doctor. She came back to the receptionist's window with instructions that I should tough it out. They wouldn't give me any triptan samples. Medication overuse meant it was my fault for having too many headaches. *Wasn't I already toughing it out?* I thought. *I had these headaches since I was thirteen years old and hadn't started taking triptans until I was in my thirties.* I don't think that's what mattered. I asked the nurse if I could speak to the doctor, but she was too busy. I'd have to make an appointment.

Desperate to control the headaches so I could function and go to work, I turned to the online black market. My searches found images of triptan pills that looked exactly like the ones I picked up at my usual pharmacy. The only difference was the cost. The ones I could order from Asia were outrageously priced, and I would have no idea if the pills were genuine or not. I was a little afraid but more embarrassed that I had to stoop that low, order pills from a seller somewhere overseas like a drug addict sneaking around to get a fix. I ordered the overpriced bottle of pills because I needed them, couldn't get the medicine any other way, had already used up all of my paid days off from work and couldn't afford unpaid sick time for an illness my employer didn't know anything about. I didn't have any more days off left to call in sick. I was out of options and money. At the end of my first year, I didn't get an offer for a permanent position. I hammered the 'for sale by owner' sign in the front yard.

**Part II**

**Prophylactic attack**

It's Just a Headache

IT WOULD ALL FIT, but I had to get it there. My eyes darted up and down, from the red needle inching up on the heat gauge to the rearview mirror. It wasn't like the Appalachian Mountains I had to pass through were real mountains, not if you asked someone from out west, like Colorado. But, the inclines were enough that the transmission strained the tiny 4-cylinder engine in the Saturn. The car already had a ton of miles on it and now, I was pulling a U-Haul trailer over 1,200 miles across the country with the leftover furniture that hadn't sold at the garage sale.

I left Eastern North Carolina late in the evening. With stops for gas, breaks and naps, the drive straight through would bring me in by afternoon the next day. The girls met me in the parking lot when I got there.

"That's it?" My oldest daughter asked surveying the small size of the trailer as I pushed down on the parking break and jumped out to give her a hug. I shook my head in agreement looking back at the tiny trailer.

"At least it won't take long to unload," I answered quietly; embarrassed as I thought back to our household belongings that filled an 18-wheeled semi-trailer packed full that had left only a year and a half before. What I had left now was downsized, but the good thing was it would fit nicely into the studio apartment I rented online ahead of time before I left North Carolina. While I didn't bring much stuff back with me to start the new research assistant position at the medical center, fifteen plus headaches every month followed me to start over, but I had better health insurance. I was broke from the abrupt sale of the house. Even though I'd sold almost every stick of furniture I owned to raise cash it didn't come close to making up the difference from what it cost to sell it. A year was not enough time for the house to appreciate in value. It didn't matter though. I was back in the same city with the girls and looking forward to starting over in the new research position. The first order of business was to get the headaches under control. I needed a doctor who could deal me some triptans.

I found a family doctor in my new insurance network, but there was no way he would agree to doling out triptans for the number of headaches I told him I was having. When I let him know that at least fifteen days of every month were headache days, he stared at me for an uncomfortable amount of time. I'm not sure if he thought I was lying, if he was trying to remember what drugs got prescribed for chronic headaches without checking my medical records on his computer or if he thought I didn't look disheveled enough to have spent at least half of my life with headaches that wouldn't go away without help. We just sat there, doctor and patient, across the room from each other and stared for too long until I broke the awkward exchange with a casual smile. Just before I started to speak, he blurted out, "Let's get you a referral to a neurologist." That's when the prophylactic attack began.

Dr. R. was close to my age. A professional, attractive, friendly and outgoing personality could have easily found her at an Ivy League medical center. Her smile and genuine interest made me afraid. My first thought was to grab my purse and run for the exit the moment I realized she was interested in what I had to say. I'd always been cattle herded through appointments; a female, age, height, weight, blood pressure, symptoms, treatment and out the door. I'd sort of grown accustomed to it and liked it that way especially since I was hiding from the headaches for so long.

"You need to be on preventative medication to bring these headaches under control," Dr. R. said in a definitive tone. It sure sounded like she was concerned with my well-being the way she said it or maybe, a lifetime of headaches had dulled my cognitive abilities to understand when someone was concerned. I agreed with everything Dr. R. said, but in my embarrassment to make a positive impression on this doctor who was treating me like a real person, I lied about how many headaches I had and how bad they were. I didn't want to describe what it was really like. I didn't want to tell her how I crawled on the floor, cried and hung my head over the toilet helpless to the pain I couldn't handle sometimes. I wanted some dignity. I wanted respect. But, I wanted to get rid of the headaches even more. I needed to get them under control. I was afraid of admitting to myself and the doctor that I feared not being able to keep the job I'd just started because the headaches got so bad at times. They'd already cost me two jobs.

I left the first appointment with a prescription for the beta blocker, metoprolol, a drug normally given to patients with high blood pressure but used off-label as a prophylactic for headaches. I didn't think it would work but was willing to give it a try. I didn't have high blood pressure, but the dose of metoprolol was low enough not to raise concern. Eager to get started, I took the first pill the same day it was filled at the pharmacy.

If I didn't have headaches, I'd never go to a medical doctor-- ever. I don't have any other health concerns. I'm in excellent physical condition. I'm not overweight. I don't have cardiac issues. I'm full of energy and stamina. In the generation I came from, we didn't complain, and if there was something wrong with us, we didn't let others to know about it. We hid our weaknesses, and that was what I'd done with these headaches all my life. Maybe that was why I didn't pay any attention to the rumblings in my stomach and assumed it was stress. I was under some pressure of expectation since I had recently started the new research fellowship at the medical center. I was building my project from the ground up and needed to generate data from experiments to write grant applications. I was starting over. If I didn't secure an independent grant, this was the end of my research career. I'd be shoved off to a corner lab in an old building to something menial like processing samples for graduate students for the rest of my career. That wasn't my plan. I had bigger goals.

My new lab had several National Institutes of Health grants which supported a full crew of technicians, graduate students, MD-PhD students, post-doctoral research fellows and senior research fellows, the latter of which was where I fell into the hierarchy. We were spread across four labs in two different buildings on the medical center campus. The bench where I worked and kept a desk was located in the north building shared with four others; a technician, graduate student, rotating M4 and an MD-PhD student. The last one in the corner past three rows, my desk was tucked in at the end of my bench. It was convenient having my desk next to where I performed experiments, so I could sit, plan and have coffee while I worked. Technically, we weren't supposed to have food or drink in the labs, but our desks were considered clean areas. That was the case until the safety inspector showed up, and then they really were clean areas. When a safety inspection was scheduled, we hid our food and drink. I usually slipped my coffee cup in between the tall, dark chemical bottles under my work bench. The inspector never checked under there.

I brought in my morning coffee and sipped on it at my desk while I planned the day's experiments. Most of the stomach rumblings would happen in the mornings after I had a bite to eat for breakfast then would settle as the day went on. Coffee seemed to help quiet the rumblings. I was standing at my corner bench gloved and in a lab coat ready to prepare some samples for an experiment that morning when the rumbling changed to a sharp and much lower intestinal cramp. I slipped off my gloves, returned to the desk and took a quick drink of coffee to see if it would help. I expected the coffee remedy would work and grabbed for another pair of gloves, stretched them on and returned to the experiment at the bench. It was a few minutes later, and I'd forgotten about the stomach pains. I was engrossed in loading a squishy blue mixture into a gel when a sudden heat wave overtook me as another sharp cramp shot from my stomach down through my bowels. There was no way I could ignore this pain. I doubled over and moved towards the desk to check and make sure I had drunk coffee and not one of the chemical reagents by mistake. Assured I had not, I leaned against the bench for support as a second cramp gripped my intestines, much harder this time. A cold sweat broke across my brow, and the gurgling of my lower bowel warned something was very wrong. I started shaking because I knew there wasn't much time. The bathrooms were outside the lab and across the building. I took a step forward, but it was too late. The forceful urge had overcome my bowels, and I could feel the warm liquid saturate the back of my pants. At that point, I thought it possible to make a run through the lab, out the door and down the hall to the ladies room to get myself cleaned up enough to wrap things up and go home but just then, the M4 rotating medical student entered the lab and rounded the corner towards his bench.

"It's a rare side-effect. Some people were sensitive," Dr. R. surmised as she listened to my brief report about the stomach discomfort I had while taking the metoprolol. We moved on. Next on the list of weapons in the prophylactic attack was one that helped stimulate the effects of Gama Amino Butyric Acid, or GABA for short. The drug was an indirect GABA agonist which meant it helped GABA do its job in the brain. The way the drug worked was not completely understood, but in people prone to seizures and in those with headaches, drugs that looked similar to GABA helped to calm the brain. A calm brain meant no headaches, presumably. I filled the prescription and started taking the GABA agonist at the lowest dose. Nothing happened for a couple of weeks, so I upped the dose like Dr. R. told me to do if there were no changes with my headaches.

It was a weeknight, and I was watching a movie on my laptop. I'd fallen asleep on the sofa and woke around 3am. I was cold and uncomfortable in the position I'd dozed off in. As I closed the laptop and placed it aside on the end table, getting ready to go to bed, a pale, blue light outside the window caught my attention. My glasses still on, I stretched my head forward to see what it was that far up above the ground illuminating the unusual glow, where no light source had ever been present before. As I tried to focus, the outline of a human figure emerged floating behind the blue light. My heart pounded. The blue glowing light and outlined human figure I could see clearly now were more than fifteen feet in the air and moving towards me. I was scared because my husband was out of town on a work trip. I had to deal with this on my own. Working up some courage, as I swung my legs from the sofa to the floor, I knew there must be some rational explanation. I jumped up and ran across the room to turn on the outside lights. The switch was next to the sliding doors.

*I'm sure I remembered to lock the doors before I fell asleep*, I confided to myself a moment before my hand swept upwards, then passed through the light switch as it dissipated into the air in a puff of smoke. *It was only a bad dream.* I sighed; relieved it was over, as I slumped against the wall. *Oh my God!* I screamed and grabbed frantically for something to hold onto to catch my fall. There was no sound from my screams as the wall disappeared, and I fell through. The next thing I knew, my body was drifting towards the human figure and blue glowing light, and the space between was closing fast. I struggled to escape, but it was useless, like trying to swim in air. As it drew nearer the air got thick like syrup until my arms and legs wouldn't move any more. I was trapped, paralyzed as the blue light source widened and encompassed my body. The blue light was cold as it overtook me. It started in my hands then moved up my arms and was working its way into my torso. In a last ditch effort to escape, I reached inside for the tiny bit of warmth that was left, keeping my core alive and mustered a final, guttural scream. That's when I woke. My glasses were on my face. The sofa throw blanket was kicked over to the side, and the pillows were on the floor.

My hands and feet were freezing and on the end table, a blue, flashing light on the laptop CD-ROM player signaled the DVD had ended and was ready to eject.

The nightmares continued until I stopped taking the GABA agonist. I didn't try any more beta blockers like metoprolol. For one, because my lab bench at work was too far away from quick access to the bathroom and second, they didn't help with my headaches. Dr. R. thought we should try tricyclics and reuptake inhibitors like amitriptyline, imipramine and bupropion (like Wellbutrin and Zyban). I followed up with her every six weeks to report any unacceptable side-effects and more importantly, to let her know if the headaches decreased, but none of these prophylactics helped. We were more interested in the anti-seizure and anti-convulsion medications, so we focused back on those even though I knew there could be bolts for the bathroom or nightmares in the near future once I started taking these kinds of drugs again.

It hit the driveway and shattered missing my big toe by less than an inch. I stepped back and assessed the broken chunks strewn across the concrete and parts that had flown into the yard as my heart raced. The force had caused a few pieces to hit my truck. I heard the dings. It was probably scratched but at the moment, my right calf hurt. Looking down, there was a trail of blood trickling its way towards my ankle. I needed to go back inside the house, get it cleaned up and check to see if any pieces were embedded, wash my hands and clean out my fingernails.

It was a loose brick in the walkway, and I was tired of tripping over it. That same loose brick had been sticking up since we'd moved into the house five years before but today, I'd had enough. When the toe of my sandal caught the edge, like it did every time I walk over it, I flew into a fit of rage. I flung my purse aside, dropped to my knees and clawed out the corners with my fingernails, now jammed full of dirt. It took a couple of tries and another kick, but when I finally got it loose enough to lift out, I raised it above my head and fired it down onto the concrete driveway. That took care of it.

I didn't know what overcame me. The sudden fits of anger took me by surprise. There was no thought ahead of time. There was only violent action. I was left to wonder what I was mad about but not this time. There was a busted brick, blood running down my calf and a dent in the fender of the truck as a stark reminder. I started taking the anti-convulsion drug, levetiracetam, thinking lucid dreams and nightmares might be the side-effect, but that didn't happen. Instead, my ability to act rationally and my fuse disappeared. I was sitting on a narrow edge, ready to explode at any moment, and I did. I was too afraid of myself to go on with this medication.

I wasn't ready to give up. I agreed with Dr. R. to try others because the headaches weren't getting any better. Beta blockers and tricyclics didn't seem to help and most of the anti-seizure drugs either caused side-effects too severe to make them useful or didn't help. That was, until the paresthesia subsided from topiramate. I remembered the pins and needles sensation from more than a dozen years before when I took an ergotamine that Anna gave me. I recognized it right away. The tingling started at the tips of my fingers, but the majority of the effect was in my face and would happen in the mornings a few hours after I took the daily dose. It was like fire ants were crawling under my skin stopping to sting every once in a while. That wasn't so bad compared to some of the strange side-effects I'd had with other drugs. I kept taking it thinking those minor tingling sensations would go away given enough time, like Dr. R. said they would.

Maybe I just forgot about the tingling and fire ants under my skin in the mornings from the topiramate. I'd taken other drugs for the six weeks trial periods where nothing happened and I'd taken so many different ones, I'd started to lose track. I didn't really notice when the tingling side-effects went away, but they did and fairly quickly. What I noticed was that the headaches changed. I was still getting the same number of them, but when I did get one, it didn't hurt quite as bad. It was as if the pain was dialed down a notch. But with that bit of relief came a loss of mental resolution. I went ahead and increased the dosage, like Dr. R. instructed after the six week follow up, but I found my upper limit of what I was able to take of the topiramate quickly when the haze of confusion made it hard to think straight.

***

I had journaled in the past. One I remembered had pink hearts on the front cover and a tiny lock on the side that secured it from prying eyes. That one was full of poetry I wrote during my teenage angst years. Later journals were scribbled with plans about what I wanted to do with my life, scientific aspirations and how I'd spend the million dollars I won from the Nobel Prize when I cured cancer. That's what crossed my mind when Dr. R. suggested I keep a journal. I already had several, but they weren't what she was looking for. I was supposed to log when I had headaches in a monthly journal, so we could get a better idea of when they occurred to see if patterns were present. The topiramate had helped to bring the intensity of headaches down, but I was still having over fifteen a month. Dr. R. thought we could add another prophylactic drug to get them under better control. We needed to see when the headaches occurred to do that.

I never had anything nice to say about the headaches except some choice words of how they had ruined perfectly good career opportunities, driven me broke and left me in pain. I didn't want to share that with the best doctor I'd ever had, so I chose a kitten calendar for my

**145**

headache journal. On days when the pain was manageable, I didn't bother to mark those, but on days when I had to take a triptan to stop the headache, I circled the date with a red Magic marker. During my monthly cycle, I marked those days in blue. It wasn't long before patterns emerged. I knew the headaches came around my monthly cycle. They'd done that since the very first one, but there were plenty of times when headaches clustered in between. I'd go into a headache phase where they would only ease up with the use of triptans back to back until the headache phase ended. I hated those because they'd last for several days at a time. Headaches phases were what used up all my monthly doses of triptans and that was a problem because belief in medication overuse headaches was firmly entrenched by then. I worried every month if I'd have enough medicine even after I broke the pills in half, which I wasn't supposed to do. During a headache phase my medicine got used up fast. I had to ration doses of triptans to work days only, like I'd done before.

It wasn't like I needed to raise my eyebrows to function normally or get my job done at work. What we tried next left me unable to move my forehead for over two months. Insurance only paid for the doctor's office visit part of the procedure. I had to cough up the cash for the medicine. It didn't hurt much. It felt like a couple of dozen bee stings. I lay back on the exam table and closed my eyes, so I wouldn't see it coming. Dr. R. was fast as she injected the front above my brow, forehead, above my ears, and I sat up as she finished with a couple in the back where my skull met my neck. The procedure was no big deal. It was supposed to act as a prophylactic along with the topiramate to help reduce the headaches. It didn't work for me. I had just as many headaches in the months that followed and was out the cash I had to pay for the expensive Botulin toxin. Dr. R. suggested we give Botox another try, but I didn't want to pay for another round of shots that wouldn't work. I was already mulling over some of my own ideas that were less expensive. It was time to take matters into my own hands.

Thirty years had passed since I first stirred up and gulped down Brewer's yeast, soy lecithin and a mix of vitamins in an effort to stop the headaches. I was ready to give home remedies another try. Modern medical prophylactics had left me with headaches and questioning if I had experimented sufficiently on my own. There was enough anecdotal information floating around on the

Internet from headache sufferers who'd tried alternative therapies and supplements with positive results. I was ready to experiment on myself.

Triptans worked and could stop a headache, but my doctors never wanted to give me the doses that matched the number of headaches I had each month. My insurance never paid for a sufficient amount of medicine to control the number of headaches I had, either. Left from this, I felt as though I was doing something wrong and was responsible for having too many headaches. I was angry at the medical approach to treating headaches, at insurance companies for their lack of foresight and at myself.

The medication overuse theory was what drove my doctors to limit supplies of medications that could help me when a headache dropped me to my knees. Their refusal to provide the number of doses that matched my headaches made me feel like a child being dealt a sip of juice before bed. It was as if I didn't know better than to spill its content all over myself or how much to drink. I knew how to treat a headache. If I caught it early enough, a dose of the triptan meant my day could go on. I could do my job and relative normalcy ensued. If I didn't have the medicine, a headache could last one or up to three days and on a few occasions, more. If it was a really bad headache, I'd have to stay home until the dizziness passed, the nausea and urge to vomit was under control and then make up some lame excuse about why I wasn't able to make it into work on time. If taking too much medicine caused headaches, then why wasn't that the case before? I'd had headaches since I was thirteen. That was dozens of years before I'd ever taken anything. I should have asked that question, but I knew what the answer was. Go home and tough it out. That was what patients with headaches were supposed to do if we were unfortunate enough to have too many headaches. I'd had enough.

I agreed with my doctors, lied and told them what they wanted to hear, so I could get the maximum amount of medicine per month my insurance would pay for then went on my way. If I knew what being an addict felt like, this was it. I felt awful having to lie to get what I needed. As the patient, my recourse was to take matters into my own hands. I'd try alternative methods to control the headaches, so I wouldn't get them in the first place. I was never fond of waking in the middle of night with my head exploding to stab myself with a needle then sit curled in the corner of the bathroom floor until the cold sweats and urge to vomit was over. It couldn't get much worse than that. I needed a better way. I needed to feel in control. I needed to stop pretending the headaches weren't that bad. They were and I was willing to experiment, even if that meant I was the pink mouse with my neck stretched out in danger of losing of my head.

I thought about the placebo effect. There was the possibility that anything I tried might work only because I believed it would. I was OK with that. As long as the headaches got better or stopped, I didn't care if it was real or placebo. If there was something safe, inexpensive, legal, easy to obtain and with few to no side-effects, I would take it or do it to stop the headaches.

I planned them out. The experiments lasted for two months each that way there was enough time to tell if anything changed. For supplements or edible therapeutic approaches, I consumed them in reasonable, safe amounts and recorded the data in the kitten calendar headache journal. In two months' time, it was easy to see from the entries if a supplement was exerting an effect compared to the red circles, which were the headache days.

I started simple. I ate dirt.

The yard was full of it. In the Midwest, windblown loess soil deposited from receding glaciers during the last ice age was packed with minerals. The problem was, finding an edible sample not contaminated with squirrel, bird, or dog urine and feces. I didn't want to eat that, so I dug down about six-inches with the shovel, which seemed like a safe zone, and collected my sample supplement.

It smelled like earthworms that come in those white, plastic containers used for fish bait. The dirt was moist, having originated from a fresh six inch zone and had a faint orange tint color. I touched the tip of my tongue to a balled up clump to explore. I could taste a hint of iron mixed with sulfur as it briefly passed over my palate. I rolled up a reasonable sized dose and popped it in my mouth, but it crumbled the moment it landed. My jaw closed ready to chew, but that wasn't going to work. The dirtball dissolved into a sandy grit with saliva as I fought back the instinctive urge to spit it out. I needed something to wash it down. It became clear to me why supplements were made into pills.

Feverfew arrived in a bottle packed into easy to swallow pills. I titrated the dose over the course of two months from the lowest to highest, as was recommend on the back label. Reasoning that the active compound might be best obtained from fresh leaves from the live plant, I went for a walk to look for it. I thought I might find the plant growing wild along the edges where the mowers didn't cut everything down. Since the Feverfew plant was considered an invasive weed where I lived, I assumed I'd find it easily but after several trips down the street to my local park and a hike through the prairie reserve turned up nothing, I ordered seeds from a vendor and planted them. I figured I'd grow the fresh stuff. I waited for the seeds to germinate, but nothing came up. I consumed the maximum dose of Feverfew pills over the course of two months but nothing changed with my headaches. I abandoned the experiment with Feverfew as failed.

I had to try magnesium. Some studies suggested that levels drop in people with chronic headaches. Whether those changes in magnesium were a cause or an effect of headaches wasn't clear, but I figured loading up on foods rich in magnesium wouldn't do any harm. After making sure there were plenty of magnesium-rich foods in the house like spinach, fish and whole grains, what was already a part of my normal diet, nothing about my headaches changed. I picked up a bottled of magnesium supplements from the drug store and took the maximum safe dose for two months. It didn't help, so I moved on to B vitamins, calcium and Ginkgo biloba. I took each of these, one at a time at their recommended dosages for two months. None changed the number or the intensity of my headaches.

I was pilfering shelves at the pharmacy searching for a new prophylactic for the headaches when I ran across capsaicin nasal spray. The active ingredient from chili peppers, capsaicin, sprayed into the sinus cavity, sets in motion pain receptors near the brain. While it was not considered a prophylactic, it was considered a treatment for a headache if used early in its progression. I was eager to give it a try a few days later when I caught a headache coming on. The tingling above my right eye was a sure sign a headache was starting. I grabbed the bottle of capsaicin nasal spray I had stashed in the medicine drawer and gave it a whirl to make sure it was mixed. I peeled off the plastic safety wrap, opened the cap and gave it a sniff. It didn't smell like hot chili pepper, so I squeeze a drop onto my finger and tasted it. It didn't taste like anything, so I squeezed the first dose up one nostril and the second dose up the other. The fire started immediately. Only my head hurt before but now, this felt like I shoved a hot branding iron up into each nostril.

*Maybe this was how it worked*, I thought as my eyes burned while I strained to read some of the fine print on the bottle. From what I was able to read before my vision blurred out, I wasn't supposed to blow my nose for the first minute while the capsaicin worked its magic. I waited more than the required minute. The burning continued. My eyes turned bloodshot red and watered and nose ran while the headache got worse. After thirty minutes, I loaded an injection, crawled into my favorite corner in the bathroom and stabbed in the shot to stop the headache. The pepper continued to burn my sinuses the rest of the night.

Snorting hot pepper didn't work for me. There were more 'fight fire with fire' strategies out there. The way to stop pain was to inflict pain, so I moved on to the Transcutaneous Electrical Nerve Stimulator, or the TENS unit for short. It was fun to play around with but the real questions were where to place the electrode pads and what milliamps setting to use. My headaches centered in the front of my head, behind my right eye (I'm a hemi headache-type). I wanted to make sure I shocked my brain in the right place. I attached the pads centered between my eyes above my nose and next to my right ear. I started the TENS unit on the lowest setting. It was paresthesia all over again and felt like the fire ants were back on my face, crawling around under my skin. It didn't feel therapeutic at all on the low setting, so I turned up the TENS unit to max. That's when I could move my ears, since I could never do that voluntarily. I wasn't willing to shave patches of my hair for the electrodes to make direct electrical contact with scalp muscles. The experimental twitches were localized to my neck, face and shoulders. Shock sessions with the TENS unit was supposed be therapeutic help for headaches, but after trying every available patch of skin where I could stick the electrode pads, it didn't decrease the number or intensity of my headaches.

For a more gentle change of pace, I tried a mind machine. These pricy devices were marketed as a way to block out external stimuli for those who practiced some forms of meditation. Comprised of a specially designed visor, headphones and control module, the device worn over the eyes and ears was supposed to alter brain waves. The visor directed beams of lights aimed at the eyes, and the headphones played sounds at different amplitudes and wavelengths programmed from the control module.

I had to save my money to buy a mind machine because it was expensive. When it finally arrived it was the hit at work. Everyone wanted to play with it. Once you slipped on the visor and headphones, picked out a program and kicked back, it was like a drug-free acid trip. The problem was these light and sound shows didn't do anything to stop my headaches. It was doubtful the mind machine altered brain waves. The concept of getting directly at the source of the problem to stop the headaches was not such a bad idea since the pain was located inside my head.

My nose itched, but I wouldn't reach up to give it a nudge. It was too late by then. I'm sure she was watching me. I tried to breathe out through my nose, ever so quietly with a snort-burst to ease the itch, but it didn't work. The tickle further intensified distracting me from the breathing pattern I was supposed to be following. *Where was I--at the slow inhale or long exhale?* I thought, slowly inching my top lip down trying to ease the irritating itch hoping she wouldn't see me. There were five of us in the session. She agreed to do all of us for a discounted price. I couldn't pass up the deal. For fifty bucks, I might be able to find the source of my headaches, but in the middle of this first hypnosis session with an itch on my nose I couldn't scratch, I didn't want her to know I wasn't under.

The therapist was a slight built older lady with dark, straight hair and a pleasant demeanor. Long, dangling necklaces with bulky beads hung around her neck color-coordinated with a black pantsuit. She welcomed us into her office that late afternoon with a smile and the usual pleasantries. Rather than a full grip handshake to greet us, she offered only the tips of her fingers brushed across our palms as if feeling for our auras. Low wattage lighting gave a relaxed ambience while the faint smell of fresh cut late summer flowers lingered in the air. The therapist allowed each of us to find our own seats in a room decorated with medium Earth tone colored chairs and loveseats arranged in a large, spread out circle. Despite the warm welcoming and the efforts to make the room comfortable, an organic skepticism set in, and my voice cracked with nervous anticipation when my turn came for an introduction.

"I'm here because I have bad headaches, and I want to get rid of them," I answered briefly, turning my head and eyes sideways to pass the introduction task on to the next person. I didn't know any of these people, so I felt safe enough to blurt that out about the headaches. The guy sitting next to me was eager to talk for the next five minutes about how he had experience with hypnosis, knew how it worked and was over excited about the immediate prospect of 'going under.' The therapist nodded and smiled with pursed lips as he introduced himself for too long then raised her slender finger towards the next person to keep the session moving along. I wasn't as enthusiastic as the rambling guy because when the session finally started, all we did was breathe. If I had known that was all there was to a hypnotic session, I might have remained home, saved the fifty bucks and taken a nap instead.

As the therapist instructed each slow inhale followed by long exhale, the nose itch intensified. It was everything I could do to resist the urge to reach up and rub the itch away. I was supposed to be under hypnosis, breathing, eyes closed and in a relaxed state of body and mind. A sudden move to rub away the irritating itch would be a sure giveaway I wasn't anywhere close to 'under.' I tried to relax and follow along with the breathing pattern, but the thirty minute session felt like it went on for hours. I was relieved when the therapist brought us up from being down under, so I could rub the dry itch away and breath normally again.

Maybe I wasn't the type that could yield to the power of suggestion or maybe my nose really did itch. Not being able to move freely wasn't relaxing, and I already knew how to breathe. Hypnosis seemed like a good idea because the headaches were inside my head, but there was the rest of my body to think about. Wishing them away under hypnosis wasn't going to work after all.

"You have to consider the whole person," she explained, finishing up the final touches to prep the room.

In the background, the hollow sound of bamboo wind chimes mixed with the scent of lavender and dried sweat as it drifted through the air. The therapist laid a hand towel and bottle of lotion on a side table then turned to switch on a small fan. "I'll give you a minute to get ready," she said, pivoting the fan away from the massage table as she slipped out of the room and quietly pulled the door closed behind her.

*Do I take off all of my clothes or leave on my underwear and bra for the massage session?* The thought spun in my mind as I hurried to get ready before she returned. She said to remove as much clothing as I was comfortable with, but I wasn't sure what that really meant. This was my first time. I hurried to undress and climbed face down on the table. A thin, white sheet pulled up to my shoulders hid my decision, but I began to doubt it and wished I had asked someone I trusted at work ahead of time what was the proper etiquette. My face was wedged in the padded O-ring face pillow which I couldn't seem to get positioned properly to keep my nose and lips from feeling like they were being squeezed out. I crept forward, careful to keep the sheet covered up to my shoulders, to prop my forehead further on the O-ring just as the therapist tapped on the door and entered the room.

"Are you comfortable?" she asked as the door clicked closed behind her. I told her I was even though my cheek bones were still wedged in awkwardly. We agreed on the massage intensity level she would apply for the session. I went with a medium pressure, therapeutic massage not knowing what that really meant.

A light breeze wafted over my exposed back as the therapist pulled the sheet down from my shoulders and tucked it in securely at my midriff. I squirmed and lifted my head just a little to de-wedge my face from the O-ring and pinched my arms tight against the tucked sheet. Then, I heard the lotion slop heavy against the insides of the plastic bottle as she shook it down, squeezed some out and rubbed it vigorously on her hands. It hadn't warmed much. Her hands were ice cold. I shivered and tensed up as the strength of her fingers chased the chill up the middle of my back. She worked her way down slowly, methodically and I felt the tension in my muscles yield to her experienced persuasion. Just as I began to think I might be able to nod off and take a nap, the deeper, therapeutic part started.

*No pain, no gain,* I kept thinking to myself as the intensity bordered my pain tolerance threshold. I forgot about my cheek bones pinched uncomfortably in the O-ring face pillow, the white sheet and if it was still pulled up covering my decision to strip naked for the massage and I wasn't cold any longer. I was about ready to tap out when she dug her elbow, deep and hard down into my trapezius, which caused my arm to go numb. I held on and answered yes when she asked if I was OK about halfway through the massage. Natural endorphins built. Pain mixed with pleasure. "You can go harder," I gasped through pinched lips after the therapist arched back from stimulating my sciatic nerve.

"You could bruise," she replied.

"That's OK." I answered. I was resolved to reach new pain-pleasure thresholds even if that meant I was black and blue afterwards. It was worth it.

The massages didn't help with my headaches, but I was hooked from the very first one and went back every month. I had both women and men. It didn't really matter as both did a good job and worked my body over until I was satisfied. I moved up to the highest level pressure and intensity massages and looked forward to the pain.

***

"The headaches follow your monthly cycle with some in between," Anna interpreted as she scanned the kitten calendar headache journal pointing to a month when I'd taken Feverfew, which didn't work. "It's hormonal with us, you know," she concluded, done with the data and looking up at me with a message I was still processing. I'd taken a long weekend and traveled out of town to visit Anna, meet her new granddaughter she'd been teeming over and get some much needed time off from work. I brought my kitten calendar headache journal along and showed it to Anna, who immediately saw what was going on.

Tucked away in rolling wheat fields insulated from the ever present hum of traffic, Anna lived in a Dutch farmhouse in the plains. A steep gravel driveway with deep ruts that continually washed out every time it rained crept up to the house from the access road. The house was a traditional two-story, with white shingled siding and had a modern sunroom addition that faced south. A line of windbreak trees stood just past the chicken pens near where Anna's husband found a mammoth thigh bone when he was raking out hay cleaning up after the chickens one day. The story was that the leghorns got hungry when he forgot to feed them and scratched so hard that they dug it up looking for bugs to eat. Outside the back door and across a crumbling concrete patio covered by a sloped roof, the vegetable garden grew on the east side shaded from the afternoon sun. My favorite place was the front yard in summer, under the canopy of a mature Sugar Maple. I loved it out there in the middle of nowhere. It was quiet, and I could think. Unlike inside the city where I lived, I could hear myself when I went to visit Anna.

We steadied the lawn chairs on the grass, adjusting them so that we were both under the shade and picked up where we left off. As Anna said of our conversations, we never needed to get reacquainted. It didn't matter if we'd not seen each other for a month or a year, there were never any formalities. It was like we knew what the other was thinking or at least Anna had a strong sense of what was important and needed talked over. I climbed on my proverbial soapbox and rambled over how important my project back in the lab was which meant I was working too many hours trying to generate data to support grant proposals. Anna pointed out the amount of time I spent at work and how much weight I had lost.

"You look gaunt," she remarked, sizing me up then looking over my head down the hill towards the gravel driveway. I had lost some weight but didn't think I was unhealthy. The demands of a research fellow aside, I was having a lot of headaches. I couldn't eat when they came on. Anna knew the headaches made us sick. I chose modern medicine to treat my headaches because it saved me precious time—that was time that I needed to pursue my career. I was seeing a neurologist taking prescription medicines and making marks in a kitten calendar headache journal. But Anna was doing better than I was. She chose the natural way and was growing her own vegetables in a garden without using artificial fertilizers or pesticides. This was what she considered medicine. She took the time to meditate and rested when she needed it. Anna no longer believed in little white pills.

A cloud of dust rose over the hill down the driveway. Mandy, Anna's daughter-in-law, pulled in. Anna's eyes lit up with anticipation as Mandy unbuckled Leah from the car seat and brought her over kicking and cooing in her carrier and sat her on the grass in front of us.

"She's beautiful and looks just like you," I remarked as Leah reached up to grab my hand when I knelt down to pick her up. Leah's tiny fingers wrapped around my thumb as I lifted her out of the carrier and sat her in my lap.

"I'll be right back," Anna said as she sprang from her chair and started walking towards Mandy, who had gone back to the car and was gathering the diaper bag. They started a conversation about when Leah had her last bottle. I settled into my seat with Leah and crossed my legs to form a secure cradle under her. She kicked her arms and legs, fast and nervously. Her eyes widened and the coos and gurgling quieted as she realized she'd been abandoned to a stranger. Agitated, her lips pursed, and it looked as if she was ready to burst out crying until she caught sight of her grandmother as she passed by on her way inside the house. Then everything changed. Gentle, upturned curves at the corners of Leah's brown eyes locked with mine imprinting a reminder of the first time I'd met Anna over thirty years before.

"This is her dinner," Anna said as she returned from the house shaking a bottle filled with an opaque colored liquid. The bottle was dripping rinse water from the kitchen sink with little bubbles visible floating on top of the liquid inside. "I made this in the juicer. I'm giving her homemade organic juices," Anna boasted, reaching over to take Leah from my lap, who eagerly took the bottle and drank. She was in good hands with her grandmother as were all of us who were close to Anna.

We hugged, said our goodbyes and I promised I wouldn't let so much time pass before I returned to visit. During the three hour drive home that late Sunday night, I thought about the data in the kitten calendar. I was playing the role of experimental scientist well. I was careful to titrate the doses of the supplements I took and record the data but I wasn't taking the time to pause and interpret what the red and blue circles meant. Anna saw the obvious relationship between the headaches and hormone cycles. It was time I formulated an experimental approach that would target the cause of the headaches.

What do men with enlarged prostate glands and premenopausal women have in common, aside from being bickering married partners at that time of their lives? It was my next approach to reduce the number of headaches I was having. I'd spent my doctoral thesis working in prostate cancer and knew a few things about the drugs used to treat it. It's important to understand the prostate gland to follow how hormones are involved.

The prostate is a small, walnut-sized gland located between the bladder and the rectum. It produces seminal fluid that helps carry sperm as part of the male reproductive system. It is located tightly squeezed between the bladder and the rectum and as a man ages, the prostate gland can enlarge due to a lifetime exposure to androgens, the male hormone better known as testosterone. If your husband spends as much time in the bathroom as you but emerges without makeup or his hair styled, it's possible he's been waiting extra time to go. His prostate may have enlarged. That's because the prostate sits on top of the urethra, which empties urine from the bladder. When the prostate enlarges it can push against, compress and make it more difficult for a man to urinate. Few men complain when something goes awry below the belt. If an over the counter remedy is available they can take privately to treat the condition, they will. In this case, there is when the enlarged prostate is benign. Saw palmetto has been in use as a treatment and has few to no side-effects. An extract from the berries of a palm tree, the pill, taken once a day, helps ease symptoms so men can go. What it does is gently relax the prostate easing pressure off the urethra. How it does this is by inhibiting enzymes involved in the hormone pathway that makes testosterone. Even though females don't have a prostate gland, we have the same enzymes that are inhibited by Saw palmetto.

Women are a complex set of hormones. The sex hormone, estrogen, is a catch-all term that describes a set of estrogen forms which includes estradiol, estriol and estrone. Each of these hormones are present at varying levels and at different stages of a woman's lifetime. We also make testosterone. While traditionally thought of as a male hormone, testosterone is what gives us energy, makes us lively and keeps us young. If hormonal imbalances occur, conditions such as premenstrual syndrome, acne and irregular periods, just to name a few of them, can result.

Four years' worth of kitten calendar headache journal entries showed the headaches clustered around my monthly cycle. I decided to test the relationship between hormone changes and headaches, so I picked up a bottle of Saw palmetto from the grocery store pharmacy aisle and took one pill per day but nothing changed after a month. I increased the dose up to two per day, and that was when I started to notice a difference. After three months' of recording how many headaches I had, a trend in the kitten calendar started to take shape.

I increased the dose of Saw Palmetto to four pills per day, a total of 640 mg of standardize extract, for another month and continued to record the number of headaches I had during that time. The higher dosage didn't decrease the headaches any further. The maximum dose response was two pills per day. Before beginning the Saw palmetto, I was having over fifteen headaches per month. After taking two pills per day, 320 mg of standardized extract, the number of headache days went down to a range of eight to twelve per month, and the best part was there were no side-effects. Saw palmetto might have been working as an enzyme inhibitor in the production of hormones that spurred headaches. I speculated that because for one, I don't have a prostate for the Saw palmetto to have been exerting its effect on and two, my terminal degree was in biochemistry. I'd done enzyme inhibition assays in the lab in the past. But, my career working in a research lab was getting ready to come to an end.

I passed a golden age. After several years as a research fellow at the medical center, time had run out. I had plenty of data from my experiments to fill the pages of grant applications, but none of them were funded. The National

Institutes of Health preferred to give funding to young scientists starting out in their careers. Once a scientist passed the age of forty, the chances of obtaining a first grant fell dramatically. Nearing my fifth decade, I was well over prime funding age and was unsuccessful at securing my own grant. It was time to move on. I left the medical center research fellow position to pursue a career in the private medical industry. My age, experience and maturity lent an upper hand in my new job, but there was frequent travel. Airplanes and headaches never mixed well, and I knew that going in, but a career in the private medical industry had more upward potential, if I could keep up. Some weeks, I was home only on weekends. While it was exciting at first, I was traveling from one end of the country to the next day after day. The headaches took their toll.

I couldn't see the traces on the computer screen in front of me. It was an ocular headache, the kind that caused my right eye to go blind, and the surgeon was at the point where he needed me to send the stimulus to test the pedicle screws. I was monitoring a back surgery, and my job was to help the surgeon make sure the metal hardware that went into the patient's spine didn't cause any problems with their nerves. Metal was conductive, just like nerves, and if metal placed in a patient's spine made contact with it, we had a problem. A patient was at risk and would experience shooting pains if the metal was placed such that it touched their nerves. That was why we made sure it was positioned carefully and strategically to stabilize the spine but didn't breach external of the bone. To ensure the pedicle was drilled out with sufficient insulating bone left intact, I needed to tell the surgeon what was on the screen in front of me, but I couldn't see it because an ocular headache had started. Ocular headaches left me blind. There was nothing I could do except wait for the shooting stars and rope-like circular spinning in my right eye to stop before my vision would return. That could take as long as 30 minutes. It was a matter of waiting it out with these ocular, blinding headaches.

The electrocautery buzzed, and a puff of smoke from burned flesh wisped up from the cauterized bleeder. The surgeons head shot up in my direction waiting for a response as he shoved the probe back into the freshly drilled pedicle. I hadn't told my employer, much less any of the surgeons I worked with, about these headaches. If my employer knew, I would have never been hired for this high stress position and if the surgeons knew, they would have never trusted the data I gave them during the countless neurosurgeries I assisted.

"Just a minute," I responded nervously as my hands scrambled across the keyboard pretending to press keys and check lead cables I couldn't see. I lied. I told the surgeon the computer system was malfunctioning, and I needed a moment to get it working. That bought me enough time to get past the ocular pressure blackout until my vision returned, so we could move on to test the pedicle depth and position the surgeon had drilled out and place the screws and hardware.

Fortunately, ocular headaches were rare. Once the blinding light show ended, that was when the pain set in. It was a real burden when a headache came on during a surgery. I couldn't exactly leave the operating room to take a triptan once a patient was exposed, and I was following their nerve traces on my computer screen. The surgeons depended on me, but the physical toll of long surgeries and frequent travel was a growing burden. When a headache came on, what I really needed was the comfort of home to take a triptan and rest while the medicine worked. That could take several hours, but I didn't have that because I couldn't leave the operating room once a case started.

Most of the surgery cases were scheduled ahead of time, so I knew where I'd be and what I'd be setup to monitor for the surgeon, but there were the add-ons and emergency cases. I was on call 24/7 for those. Vern, as I'll call him for privacy purposes, was one of those emergency add-on cases. He fell one morning in his kitchen. It wasn't a big deal except that Vern was in his seventies, frail and the fall left him motionless on the floor. Triage in the emergency department suggested a spinal cord injury, and the follow up MRI showed a break in his spine. The complications for Vern were that he came with a crash cart load of comorbidities. He had hypertension, diabetes, was overweight and now, a spinal injury that left him unable to control his diaphragm to move air in and out of his lungs.

I was scheduled to monitor two routine cases that day with one of my favorite surgeons. We'd been through dozens of cases together, and I was comfortable with his style of handling staff in the operating room. We were in the middle of the second case when the call came in to add-on Vern. I'd need to hook him up for monitoring to see what nerve functions he had left. The second case wrapped up, and I moved my equipment to a prepped operating room to get setup for Vern. I needed to monitor him for sensory and motor functions, to see if he could feel or move any of his extremities below the level of where the break in his spine occurred. He didn't need to be awake for any of that. He shouldn't be because I'd be poking needles into him to pick up those tiny nerve impulses and reading the traces on a computer screen to see if his nerves worked or not.

The circulating nurse buzzed into the operating room with an oversized manila envelope in her hand. She flipped it open and pulled out a film then studied the fine print on the bottom corner. Satisfied the MRI image belonged to Vern, she clipped it onto the overhead lightbox located above where I had setup my equipment. Once I finished the cleaning protocol for the cables and leads from the previous case, I began preparations for Vern. I secured the lead cables onto the Jackson table, tucking them out of the way of the surgeon and anesthesiologist. Vern would be prone positioned for his surgery, so I wrapped the cables such that they wouldn't jostle lose when we turned Vern over onto his belly for the operation.

I planned to get the equipment setup then run over to the cafeteria to grab a sandwich and cram it down before heading to pre-op holding to check Vern's health stats so I could get an idea of what I was up against before the operation started. The cup of coffee and banana I had for breakfast at 6am that morning was not going to hold me through a third case. It was already past 3pm. My stomach was starting to hurt, and a dull throb on the right side of my head threatened of an oncoming headache. I was still running system checks on the equipment when the operating room doors flung open.

The bed rumbled in with a urine collection bag clipped on the side rail, a portable ventilator hissing and an IV pole in tow. Vern had arrived. He had been intubated in the emergency room which was a bad sign as that meant he was unable to breathe on his own. The chief anesthesiologist usually performed or supervised the intubation in the operating room before surgery started. But, that was good news for me. Vern was already under. I could get him hooked up and start poking the needles in right away. I didn't have wait until anesthesia went through the time consuming stages of going under. I grabbed the electrode setup I strung together for his case. He needed them placed from head to toe. I popped in the lower sets first then moved up. There was already an IV in one of Vern's arms, but the anesthesiologist liked to have an extra vein in the other arm, for an emergency backup IV, so I waited to place electrodes needles in the arms until last and moved on up to Vern's head.

Careful not to jar the endotracheal tube, I pulled up gently on the elastic band holding the surgical cap around Vern's head. Patches of white, wiry strands of hair jutted out onto his pasty forehead as I jabbed electrode needles under the skin of his scalp. There wasn't much fat. The needles scraped against bone, though I tried to pinch and pull upward to grab enough skin for the needles to sink into, so they'd have something around them to detect the nerve traces. With the scalp electrodes in, I leaned back for a moments pause to visually recheck their proper pattern then stretched the surgical cap over his head, careful to tuck the strands of his hair in with the wires. Anesthesia had placed their backup IV by then, so I stabbed the remaining electrodes in his arms, then double and triple checked Vern's electrode placement to make sure they were secured for positioning. I didn't want any to come loose when we flipped him over.

"One, two, three," the anesthesiologist counted off as two nurses, a scrub technician, the physician's assistant and I maneuvered in sync and rolled Vern from the hospital bed onto the Jackson table at the count of three. I immediately began checking electrodes, running my fingers quickly over the tapped down leads protruding out of Vern's body to feel if any had jarred loose. They felt secured as I traced the cables and tucked overhangs before I ran back to the computer, in a hurry to start the traces to make sure current was running. Once Vern was draped and the sterile scrub began, I wouldn't be able to access the electrodes again.

The surgeon entered the room, scrubbed in with his arms held up and ready for the circulating nurse to don his sterile gown. As he stepped into the surgical field, he asked for the light box turned on under the MRI image. I reached behind me and flipped the switch. The light illuminated the full extent of Vern's injury and showed an unstable fracture with dislocation-- one of the worst types of breaks that can happen to the spine.

"What's he got?" The surgeon asked as he reached up and slid the sterile grip on the overhead surgical light head post, positioning the height and angle for the surgery.

"I'll check his motor functions now," I replied as I charged up current preparing to send a jolt into Vern's skull. The stimulus sent an electrical current through the wires I had plugged into Vern's head, across the insulating bone of his skull and into the motor center of his brain. Vern's brain picked up the electrical stimulus, processed the signal and further sent it down his spinal cord. This was the way to test the integrity of his spinal cord. I had electrodes positioned in Vern, all the needles I poked into his arms and legs, to measure if they received that signal, which showed up as traces on my computer screen. If the electrical signal was able to travel the length of the spinal cord freely, Vern's arm and leg muscles would twitch. They did, although weak, which meant Vern might have had some function in his arms and legs despite that his spinal cord was severely damaged. I charged up again and sent a couple of more jolts into Vern's skull, to make sure I had good readings, recorded baselines, and the surgeon started the exposure a little after 5:30pm.

Opening a patient's layers of skin, muscle and tissue to expose the area to fix a problem could often take a while, depending on what was being exposed and the skill of the surgeon. In Vern's case, keeping him under anesthesia was the greatest risk threatening his life at the moment. The complexity of the surgery was not going to shorten the time he would be under. It was up to the anesthesiologist to make sure Vern remained alive, stable and relaxed while the surgeon fixed his broken spine. The problem was that the added medications to keep Vern under and relaxed made it more difficult to monitor what his nerves were doing. We were trying to save any nerve function Vern may have had left. As 8pm rolled by, between the splitting headache and growling stomach, I watched Vern's traces as his spinal column was finally exposed.

"Has anything changed?" The surgeon asked as he assessed the damage now visible under the retractors. I charged up current and sent another jolt into Vern's skull, the same as before, and overlaid it to the baselines I'd established prior to when exposure started.

"I'm not picking up anything in the legs," I reported back as the surgeon focused his attention to the MRI image above my head on the lightbox. Vern had lost some ground since we started. That loss could have been from the positioning, anesthesia or during the long exposure. The surgeon knew all those things. The operation to fix the injury came with risks. Vern's spine broke in half such that the weight of his upper body displaced the spinal column and severed his spinal cord. Blunt force against weak bone in the fall caused the broken spinal column to overlap itself and shift several centimeters. Even though the spinal cord itself would never heal, it was necessary to realign the bones, end to end, like the spine was before it broke in half. Metal rods and screws would be placed along the sides to hold it secured while the bones healed. But, realignment was no easy task. After another hour passed, the surgeon couldn't get the spine adjusted from the exposure site. He stepped back, removed his blood smeared gloves and slung them across the room into the biohazard container.

"Keep his shoulders from sliding up," He instructed the room nurse as he approached Vern's head, leaned down and locked his forearms firmly on both sides in a vice-like grip and started pulling forward. "C-arm!" The surgeon yelled out for the radiology technician to shoot an x-ray to see if his efforts had moved Vern's spine. The image quickly appeared on the screen. The bones hadn't budged. Determined, the surgeon took in a deep breath and tightened his grip around Vern's head again. He pulled harder as the C-arm continued to shoot x-rays to guide his efforts. Image after image followed each x-ray, but his spine refused to move.

Vern's blood pressure suddenly spiked dangerously high. He'd been under for more than six hours, and his spine was not aligned. The forceful tugging on his head as an alternative method was more than his body could take. The surgeon loosened his grip and left the operating room to scrub in again while anesthesia gave Vern medicine to get his blood pressure under control.

"What's it look like now?" The surgeon asked as he reentered, arms held up dripping from the fresh scrub, as the circulator donned his new sterile gown and gloves. I charged up current and sent another jolt into Vern's skull. The traces on my computer screen were flat. I checked, again, to make sure the system controls worked. The wires were all connected, so I charged up current yet again and sent another jolt into Vern's skull to make absolutely sure. Nothing came back.

"I'm not receiving any signals below the shoulders," I reported as the surgeon approached the operating table and prepared to stabilize Vern's spine, overlapped as it was.

We finished after midnight. Vern was wheeled out destined to remain on a ventilator for the three days he would live after the surgery. I left the operating room with a full blown headache for the airport. My next case was 900 miles away scheduled to start first thing the following morning. I was dead tired and hungry sitting in the terminal waiting for the flight to board. The triptan I'd taken was starting to kick in, but my stomach hurt because I hadn't eaten in almost 24 hours. I found a vending machine and dropped in the handful of quarters for the overpriced, stale granola bar and bottle of water. Looking forward to the hour and a half of sleep I'd get on the redeye flight once we boarded, I pulled out my laptop and started writing the resignation letter. I'd send it in to my boss in a couple of days once I got back home.

***

An overnight freeze had taken my garden annuals that late September. I'd saved a few potted plants that were sitting out on the deck, and squeezed them onto a shelf, so they could get sun through the window. The attached four season sunroom faced south, west and north and was partially shaded by a Norway maple. Foliage blocked out the blistering sun during summer months but in winter, enough light came through to warm the room comfortably. A Bamboo palm center pieced the entry with fronds brushed against the ceiling. Along the sides and against the double paned energy efficient windows perennial exotics grew. A lemon, tangerine and a struggling avocado tree I had sprouted from seed were good reminders, on a cold day, of why I'd built the room in the first place. A sofa was parked against the west windows, faced into the sunroom and I placed an Earth toned deep shag throw rug in front of the sofa to make the room barefoot comfortable. When I needed a getaway from work, I camped on the sofa surrounded by my plants. My office was only a few steps away around the corner in the other room.

It was midafternoon and I'd taken a short break to sit in the sunroom. The sun was out. It was a deep blue cold day outside with a crisp hue forewarning of an early fall. I settled into comfortable on the sofa to read a few chapters of my book when the phone rang. It was Mandy.

"Is this Christy?" The voice mumbled, barely audible on the other end of the line. I didn't know who it was at first because I'd never talked to Mandy on the phone before. She was Anna's daughter-in-law, but I'd only ever saw or spoke to her when I went to visit. I wasn't familiar with the sound of her voice especially the low tone she was using.

"It's Anna," her voice paused. "She passed away last night in her sleep," Mandy continued, her voice trembling with the difficulty of getting the words out.

"What?" I blurted out as if I hadn't heard her correctly. The conversation paused, and a silence settled in between us for what seemed like several minutes. It was taking me some time to process what Mandy had just said.

"She's gone," Mandy finished.

I entered immediate denial. This couldn't be true. Anna was too young. I'd just visited her two months before, and she was fine. People don't die suddenly like that, I thought as my mind struggled to make sense of what I'd just heard.

My eyes searched past the glass windows to find something to say as the deep blue disappeared outside. The exotic plants on both sides of me began to fade-- they weren't green, gray or black. They no longer existed. Then, the weight of gravity settled in and I gathered myself to answer Mandy.

"I'll call you back," my voice choked out the words as I hung up and dropped the phone, its fall cushioned in the deep nap of the shag carpet throw rug.

I stumbled outside barefoot and in a daze to sit next to the pergola. My husband and I had built it ourselves the prior spring. We planted a wisteria at the base lattice, and the vines had made good growth progress that first season. They had reached the top and were spread across the girth, but the leaves had dropped with the early freeze. Only the twisted vines remained.

I sat on the concrete next to the pergola and raised my head up towards the dormant vines. My eyes followed the counterclockwise braids as they grasped each other and the lattice for support. If this was just a bad dream, I'd wake up once the cold from the concrete below me sunk in and the wind hit me in the face. I took in slow, metered breaths then something moved and caught my attention. On the top corner of the pergola, a hummingbird appeared. It hovered and assessed my presence, seemingly not afraid I had encroached on its space. It looked like a female from the muted plumage. After a moment, she skirted away then returned a few feet lower in front of the pergola and within my reaching distance.

*What did a hummingbird want on such a cold day?* I thought as she flew past my face and I turned to track her movement. The wisteria hadn't made any flowers, and there weren't any others in bloom as we were nearing the fall season. She returned and fluttered to a midair stop. Her tiny, black dots eyes caught and fixated on mine. Gentle, upturned curves blended with the crown of her plumage. It was clearly a female. I lifted my hand to reach up and then, back to her instinctive senses, she turned and flirted away. Her fear brought mine to surface and the cold that had, by then, sunk into my bones. I started to shiver uncontrollably.

***

I unscrewed the lid and shook out two Saw palmetto gel caps then grabbed for the prescription bottle of topiramate. The small, round, white, 100 mg pill rolled out and into my palm. I swallowed them down with a sip of water then headed over to my desk to check work emails. I sat down and keyed in my username and password to login to the server. Three messages had arrived since late afternoon. I'd open and read these to see what needed done. It made mornings start easier if I triaged problems before bed. As I clicked to open the first email and waited for it to load, I leaned forward in my chair and reached up to close the blinds.

My desk faced west against a window overlooking the porch lined with tall, evergreen privet shrubs. To the southwest quarter of the yard, foliage from a Sugar Maple cast a tall shadow and provided shade in late afternoon summers. Further back, a young Blue ice cypress demarked a boundary between mine and the neighbor's property lines. Across the driveway and tucked to the north, a Cherry blossom sat ornamental and out of place. During the daytime, Mockingbirds, Blue jays and Northern

Cardinals skirted between the trees just enough to keep the quiet cul-de-sac lively with their business traffic.

I took over the dining room and converted it to an office. The ten by twelve foot room fit my desk, bookshelves, two computers, a printer and even some space left over for a couch if I needed to lie down when a headache came on. That was why I exited the daily commute to the outside world to work in the first place. It was much easier to manage a day at work through a headache on my own terms from home especially, since my employer didn't know I had them. I made up my own missing time gaps at work as a telecommuter. Telecommuting exploded in popularity when companies realized that employees could be productive, trusted and a larger talent pool recruited since location was no longer a consideration for employment. What employers didn't know was that some of us hid a few things from them.

I became a full-time telecommuter after I resigned my position in private medical. I already had a part-time gig on the side, making extra money trying to pay off my student loans, so I picked up more contracts to keep me busy every day of the week. The first couple of years working from home were the best. I was excited about taking on multiple contracts and setting my own work schedule. I liked the feeling of self-control that gave me and put it to good use. Over productivity was the driving force. I was getting daily work and projects completed on or before schedule, and then jumping into home chores by 9am with time to spare. I started and finished side projects—from organizing cluttered closets to cleaning dusty baseboards, plus every other menial project I could come up with. I learned how to plant and tend a garden, in honor of Anna, but none of these staved off the isolation or made the headaches any less frequent. The worst part was that I missed the daily interaction with real people. The tradeoff was that I was able to successfully hide headaches from my employers and colleagues that existed only as names in front of me on a computer screen.

"You're a garden variety," Dr. B. stated as he flipped the folder open and began his scan of my patient file peering up to examine me, briefly, over his heavy framed glasses. A short, stocky man dressed in green scrubs, he sat on a stool next to the patient exam table, which served to hold my files, while I sat across the room in a chair. Customary of most doctors I'd had over the years, a physical examination was not performed. I assumed my medical file indicated good news. I must have had stable blood pressure, healthy body weight and maybe I looked OK, for that day, even though I'd not dyed my hair in over a year and didn't bother to put on any makeup that morning before I rushed out the door to make it to the appointment on time. As he continued to thumb through the pages of my patient file, I wondered if he planned to head over to the hospital after our appointment given his attire in scrubs, but I didn't ask. I also didn't mention crawling on the floor, the tears, sitting curled up in the bathroom corner and the dry heaves-type of headaches I had. He didn't ask. A doctor of his experience had heard plenty of these kinds of stories over the course of his career. Dr. B. glanced up at me again as he flipped on through my file. I smiled politely, preserving my dignity instead.

Dr. B. had entered medical school around the time I was born. I knew that because I looked up his professional profile to find the date of his residency. I suspected from the first appointment our doctor-patient relationship would be short lived, because he was nearing retirement age, but I chose to drive the extra distance to his office from my home. With his many years of experience, I secretly hoped he might have some age-old approach that could help me.

My concern was my age, the fact the headaches weren't getting any better and the one I might never wake from. They were harder to deal with now that I was older, but I didn't mention any of that. My life was no more or less stressful than anyone else and I didn't want to complain. I was otherwise healthy, normal weight, and took good care of my body. The best I could do with my efforts was to bring the headaches down to eight to twelve per month. Dr. B. assured me that they would decrease or resolve with menopause.

*What about now?* I wanted to ask, but I didn't. I worried instead as he closed my folder then pulled the prescription pad out of his pocket. He scribbled my standard prescriptions, peeled the rectangular squares off the book then stretched his arm out and motioned for me to take them.

"I'll see you again in six months," he instructed as I stood and reached over to accept the papers. I paused for a moment to look at the illegible handwriting then glanced down at Dr. B., who had reopened my folder and was taking some last minute notes. "The receptionist will set your next appointment up front," he said with a tone of irritation in his voice, sensing that my hesitation meant that I might want to ask a question. I nodded and smiled, thanked the doctor for his time, then shoved the prescriptions in my purse and moved quickly towards the door as the impatience in his voice sent me on my way. I'd learned from experience that it was best to agree and oblige. That was the best way to get the medicine I needed.

## EPILOGUE

I MADE A CONSCIOUS decision to use the term headache instead of migraine in this book. It would have been just as easy to interchange the two words or use the word migraine exclusively throughout. It was understood that migraine was a type of headache and even this could be further divided into subtypes. Rather than get into specific medical details about headaches and migraines, I chose to share the human experience. This was what impacted my life.

I don't remember any traumatic events from childhood. I was a happy child. I had a normal upbringing, no significant injuries, no allergies and no physical health concerns. The first headache I experienced at the age of thirteen when I passed out in the hallway at school raised little concern from my parents because I was otherwise healthy. I hid the headaches afterwards, so they never raised the issue again. The curious looks from my mother as I sat in the back seat of the car on the ride home from school gripped in pain from the first one weren't from distrust, but suspicions that I had them, too.

Hiding the headaches was a lifelong habit. In the era I grew up in, we didn't let others know about what was wrong with us. I didn't want the debilitating headaches to define me since the first one left suspicions during an impressionable time in my life. I was in my early teens, recently moved across the country, and was involved in a relationship triangle. I was never the same after the first headache. I was a good kid, smart, dedicated and with future plans that changed the day I stumbled out of class and collapsed in the hallway. But, Jerry and Sissy were doubtful. After my family moved back to Florida, I sent letters, but Jerry never wrote or called. Years later, I passed through Knoxville on my way to a meeting on the East coast. I booked the flight so I'd have a day layover, rented a car and drove to Andes Ridge. I used the TomTom GPS to find my way since I'd never driven there before. When I lived on Andes Ridge Road, I was too young to drive. It was either my parents or Kara at the wheel navigating the narrow, winding roads. I quickly realized how treacherous it was, a flatlander trying to find their way back to a memory in the Appalachian Mountains.

The red dot on the TomTom indicated I had arrived. I pulled in sideways in front of the restaurant. The building looked smaller than I had remembered it, but the bell atop the door was still visible through the window. Around the side, a fence had been constructed blocking access to the alley that led to my former home. I shut off the engine and sat for a moment as doubt started to build. Had I made the right decision to come back and what would I ask? *Hi, I'm lost, where's Jerry?* Andes Ridge was a small town. After more than twenty years, I was a city stranger passing through. Would anyone remember the thirteen year old who frequented years before to play pool, buy peanuts and soda?

I saw the blinds move as someone peeked out the window of the restaurant, curious to see who was in the car in the parking lot. I grabbed my cell phone and started a pretend conversation to stall for more time to think my decision over. *What if Jerry was married?* The uncomfortable thought burned in my mind. Surely, he was by now. Maybe I could find Kara or Sissy, but I was never close friends with them. Jerry never wrote or called, after all these years had passed. He must have moved on.

My hand tired of holding the phone to my ear in the fake conversation. The curious looks out of the restaurant window advanced to an older woman, a crew coffee regular, who came outside to check nothing on the front door but more likely get a better look at me. I glanced up to acknowledge the woman, smiled and waved in a friendly gesture. After a quick check of the building side where the fence blocked the alley, she returned inside. My eyes followed her to the blocked alley, where I found resolve. I started the car and backed up to leave. It was time to move on.

Failure was the best teacher. I learned more from mistakes than from successes. The experiments to manage the headaches were like that. My failures showed what didn't work. What was left, untried and untested must have held the keys to the relief I was looking for. That was the reasoning I followed for years on end. There were more experiments, herbal remedies, approaches and therapies than I had time to describe. Some had no effect, others made me ill and some, it was too embarrassing to admit I tried. Pain leads one onto strange paths of desperation. In nearly all experiments, I stayed with the plan until there was a verdict on whether or not the headaches were decreased. In nearly all of the experiments, they were not.

There are millions of us out there who suffer from chronic headaches. They impact our lives in every way imaginable. For the majority of us, there is no cure and in this book, I offered none. This book shared with you the human side, my experience. I chose to hide these debilitating headaches from everyone save for only those closest to me. It was Anna, who I owed a lifetime of debt for her wisdom and guidance. We shared a common bond, a start as single women working our way through college raising children, fierce independence, chronic headaches we tried to manage and a genuine friendship that ended too soon.

It was like any other on the last day of Anna's life. She had things to get done, plans made, but a headache got in the way. She'd finished some laundry and hung it outside for a fresh air dry that late afternoon. Her head hurt, so she told her husband she was going inside to lie down for a while on the sofa in the living room. Anna appeared comfortable and asleep when her husband checked on her later that evening. He left her peacefully overnight.

Anna didn't like to take medicines. She took matters into her own hands. Like the rest of us, modern prophylactics were expensive, came with too many side-effects or didn't work. Headache rescue medicines had similar problems. Insurance didn't provide adequately to pay for enough doses and after a lifetime of being blamed for having too many headaches, she'd had enough.

She'd gone all natural and it was working for her. She was active, slim, ate a clean, vegan diet and took good care of herself. Her belief was that our bodies could heal if we gave them proper nutrition, rest and time. Despite all her efforts, she still had headaches. When they came, she went to lie down and waited them out. It was just a matter of time and putting up with the pain until they were over.

Anna's husband knew something was amiss when she wasn't up before he was the next morning. She was always awake before sunrise, busy about the house making breakfast but this morning, it was quite-- too quiet. The clothes hung heavy and wet with morning dew on the line outside. There weren't any vegetables laid out for the juicer. The morning sun peeked in the window of the living room as Anna lay still. Sometime during the night, her pain ended for the last time.

It's Just a Headache

C.A. Rothermund-Franklin is an Associate Professor of Science Technology Engineering and Math. She facilitates courses at Boston University Metropolitan College for the Undergraduate Degree Completion Program. As a published author of multiple peer-reviewed scientific studies in cancer research, she has traveled nationally and internationally to give presentations, earned honor and leadership awards all while mastering the art of hiding chronic migraine headaches for over forty years. She lives in the TN Valley with her husband David.

www.ingramcontent.com/pod-product-compliance
Lightning Source LLC
Chambersburg PA
CBHW060451280326
41933CB00014B/2726